Low-Grade Glioma

Editors

GUY M. MCKHANN
HUGUES DUFFAU

NEUROSURGERY
CLINICS OF NORTH AMERICA

www.neurosurgery.theclinics.com

Consulting Editors
RUSSELL R. LONSER
DANIEL K. RESNICK

January 2019 • Volume 30 • Number 1

ELSEVIER

1600 John F. Kennedy Boulevard • Suite 1800 • Philadelphia, Pennsylvania, 19103-2899

http://www.theclinics.com

NEUROSURGERY CLINICS OF NORTH AMERICA Volume 30, Number 1
January 2019 ISSN 1042-3680, ISBN-13: 978-0-323-65501-9

Editor: Stacy Eastman
Developmental Editor: Laura Fisher

Neurosurgery Clinics of North America (ISSN 1042-3680) is published quarterly by Elsevier Inc., 360 Park Avenue South, New York, NY 10010-1710. Months of issue are January, April, July, and October. Business and Editorial Offices: 1000 John F. Kennedy Blvd., Suite 1800, Philadelphia, PA 19103-2899. Customer Service Office: 11830 Westline Industrial Drive, St. Louis, MO 63146. Periodicals postage paid at New York, NY, and additional mailing offices. Subscription prices are $430.00 per year (US individuals), $748.00 per year (US institutions), $470.00 per year (Canadian individuals), $928.00 per year (Canadian institutions), $513.00 per year (international individuals), $928.00 per year (international institutions), $100.00 per year (US students), and $255.00 per year (international and Canadian students). International air speed delivery is included in all *Clinics* subscription prices. All prices are subject to change without notice. **POSTMASTER:** Send address changes to *Neurosurgery Clinics of North America*, Elsevier Periodicals Customer Service, 11830 Westline Industrial Drive, St. Louis, MO 63146. **Customer Service: 1-800-654-2452 (US and Canada). From outside the US and Canada, call: 1-314-453-7041. Fax: 1-314-453-5170. E-mail: JournalsCustomerService-usa@elsevier.com (for print support) and journalsonlinesupport-usa@elsevier.com (for online support).**

Reprints. For copies of 100 or more, of articles in this publication, please contact the Commercial Reprints Department, Elsevier Inc., 360 Park Avenue South, New York, NY 10010-1710. Tel. 212-633-3874; Fax: 212-633-3820; E-mail: reprints@elsevier.com.

Neurosurgery Clinics of North America is covered in *MEDLINE/PubMed (Index Medicus), EMBASE/Excerpta Medica, and Current Contents/Clinical Medicine (CC/CM).*

Contributors

CONSULTING EDITORS

RUSSELL R. LONSER, MD
Professor and Chair, Department of
Neurological Surgery, The Ohio State
University Wexner Medical Center, Columbus,
Ohio, USA

DANIEL K. RESNICK, MD, MS
Professor and Vice Chairman, Program
Director, Department of Neurosurgery,
University of Wisconsin-Madison School of
Medicine and Public Health, Madison,
Wisconsin, USA

EDITORS

GUY M. McKHANN, MD
Director of Brain Mapping for Tumors and
Epilepsy, Department of Neurological Surgery,
Columbia University Medical Center/New York
Presbyterian Hospital, New York, New York,
USA

HUGUES DUFFAU, MD, PhD
Department of Neurosurgery, Gui de Chauliac
Hospital, Montpellier University Medical
Center, Montpellier, France; Institute for
Neuroscience of Montpellier, INSERM U1051,
Team "Plasticity of Central Nervous System,
Human Stem Cells and Glial Tumors," Saint
Eloi Hospital, Montpellier University Medical
Center, Montpellier, France

AUTHORS

LUC BAUCHET, MD, PhD
Praticien Hospitalier, Department of
Neurosurgery, Gui de Chauliac Hospital,
Montpellier University Medical Center,
Montpellier, France; Institute for Neuroscience
of Montpellier, INSERM U1051, Team
"Plasticity of Central Nervous System, Human
Stem Cells and Glial Tumors," Saint Eloi
Hospital, Montpellier University Medical
Center, Montpellier, France

LORENZO BELLO, MD
Unit of Neurosurgical Oncology, Department of
Hematology and Hemato-Oncology Università
degli Studi di Milano, Neurosurgical Oncology,
Humanitas Research Hospital, IRCCS,
Rozzano, Italy

MITCHEL S. BERGER, MD
Professor and Chair, Department of
Neurological Surgery, Director, Brain Tumor
Center, University of California San Francisco,
San Francisco, California, USA

DEVIN BREADY, BS
Department of Neurosurgery, NYU School of
Medicine, New York, New York, USA

RICHARD W. BYRNE, MD
Department of Neurosurgery, Rush University
Medical Center, Chicago, Illinois, USA

DANIEL P. CAHILL, MD, PhD
Department of Neurosurgery, Massachusetts
General Hospital, Boston, Massachusetts,
USA

PETER CANOLL, MD, PhD
Professor, Department of Pathology and Cell
Biology, Director of Neuropathology, Columbia
University, Columbia University Medical
Center, Irving Cancer Research Center,
New York, New York, USA

VICTORIA E. CLARK, MD, PhD
Department of Neurosurgery, Massachusetts
General Hospital, Boston, Massachusetts,
USA

LAURA E. DONOVAN, MD
Neuro-Oncology Fellow, Departments of
Neurology, Columbia University Irving
Medical Center, Weill Cornell Medicine,
NewYork-Presbyterian Hospital, New York,
New York, USA

HUGUES DUFFAU, MD, PhD
Department of Neurosurgery, Gui de Chauliac
Hospital, Montpellier University Medical
Center, Montpellier, France; Institute for
Neuroscience of Montpellier, INSERM U1051,
Team "Plasticity of Central Nervous System,
Human Stem Cells and Glial Tumors," Saint
Eloi Hospital, Montpellier University Medical
Center, Montpellier, France

LUCA FORNIA, PhD
Laboratory of Motor Control, Department of
Medical Biotechnologies and Translational
Medicine, Università degli Studi di Milano,
Humanitas Research Hospital, IRCCS, Milano,
Italy

GUILLAUME HERBET, PhD
Department of Neurosurgery, Montpellier
University Medical Center, Institute for
Neuroscience of Montpellier, Saint-Eloi
Hospital, INSERM U1051, University of
Montpellier, Montpellier, France

SHAWN L. HERVEY-JUMPER, MD
Associate Professor, Department of
Neurological Surgery, University of California
San Francisco, San Francisco, California,
USA

TODD HOLLON, MD
Department of Neurosurgery, University of
Michigan, Ann Arbor, Michigan, USA

ASGEIR S. JAKOLA, MD, PhD
Institute of Neuroscience and Physiology,
Sahlgrenska Academy, Department of
Neurosurgery, Sahlgrenska University Hospital,
Gothenburg, Sweden; Department of
Neurosurgery, St. Olavs Hospital, Trondheim,
Norway

ANDREW B. LASSMAN, MS, MD
John Harris Associate Professor of Neurology,
Chief of Neuro-oncology, Department of
Neurology, Medical Director, Clinical Protocol
Data & Management Office, Herbert Irving
Cancer Comprehensive Cancer Center,
Columbia University Irving Medical Center,
NewYork-Presbyterian Hospital, New York,
New York, USA

GUY M. McKHANN, MD
Director of Brain Mapping for Tumors and
Epilepsy, Department of Neurological Surgery,
Columbia University Medical Center/New York
Presbyterian Hospital, New York, New York,
USA

MINESH P. MEHTA, MD
Deputy Director, Miami Cancer Institute,
Baptist Hospital, Miami, Florida, USA

SYLVIE MORITZ-GASSER, PhD
Department of Neurosurgery, Montpellier
University Medical Center, Institute for
Neuroscience of Montpellier, Saint-Eloi
Hospital, INSERM U1051, University of
Montpellier, Montpellier, France

MARCO CONTI NIBALI, MD
Unit of Neurosurgical Oncology, Department of
Hematology and Hemato-Oncology Università
degli Studi di Milano, Neurosurgical Oncology,
Humanitas Research Hospital, IRCCS,
Rozzano, Milano, Italy

DANIEL ORRINGER, MD
Department of Neurosurgery, University of
Michigan, Ann Arbor, Michigan, USA

QUINN T. OSTROM, PhD, MPH
Postdoctoral Associate, Department of
Medicine, Section of Epidemiology and
Population Sciences, Dan Duncan
Comprehensive Cancer Center, Baylor College
of Medicine, Houston, Texas, USA

JOHAN PALLUD, MD, PhD
Department of Neurosurgery, Sainte-Anne
Hospital, Paris Descartes University, Sorbonne
Paris Cité, Paris, France; Réseau d'Etude des
Gliomes, REG, Groland, France; Inserm, U894,
Centre Psychiatrie et Neurosciences, Paris,
France

DIMITRIS G. PLACANTONAKIS, MD, PhD
Department of Neurosurgery, Kimmel
Center for Stem Cell Biology, Laura and
Isaac Perlmutter Cancer Center,
Neuroscience Institute, Brain Tumor Center,
NYU School of Medicine, New York, New York,
USA

MARCO ROSSI, MD
Unit of Neurosurgical Oncology, Department of
Hematology and Hemato-Oncology Università
degli Studi di Milano, Neurosurgical Oncology,
Humanitas Research Hospital, IRCCS,
Rozzano, Milano, Italy

NADER SANAI, MD, FAANS, FACS
J.N. Harber Professor of Neurological Surgery,
Director, Division of Neurosurgical Oncology,
Director, Ivy Brain Tumor Center, Barrow
Neurological Institute, Phoenix, Arizona, USA

SEPEHR SANI, MD
Department of Neurosurgery, Rush University
Medical Center, Chicago, Illinois, USA

ANJA SMITS, MD, PhD
Institute of Neuroscience and Physiology,
Sahlgrenska Academy, Gothenburg, Sweden;
Department of Neuroscience, Section of
Neurology, Uppsala University, Uppsala,
Sweden

WALTER STUMMER, Prof Dr Med
Department of Neurosurgery,
University Hospital of Münster, Münster,
Germany

ERIC SUERO MOLINA, MBA, Dr Med
Department of Neurosurgery, University
Hospital of Münster, Münster, Germany

DANIELA TORRES, PhD
Department of Pathology and Cell
Biology, Columbia University, Columbia
University Medical Center, Irving Cancer
Research Center, New York, New York,
USA

TONY J.C. WANG, MD
Associate Professor, Department of
Radiation Oncology, Herbert Irving
Comprehensive Cancer Center, Columbia
University Medical Center, New York,
New York, USA

Contents

Epidemiology, Pathophysiology, and Classification

Incidence, prevalence, and survival for diffuse low-grade gliomas and diffuse anaplastic gliomas (including grade II and grade III astrocytomas and oligodendrogliomas) varies by histologic type, age at diagnosis, sex, and race/ethnicity. Significant progress has been made in identifying potential risk factors for glioma, although more research is warranted. The strongest risk factors that have been identified thus far include allergies/atopic disease, ionizing radiation, and heritable genetic factors. Further analysis of large, multicenter epidemiologic studies, and well-annotated "omic" datasets, can potentially lead to further understanding of the relationship between gene and environment in the process of brain tumor development.

Advances in genome sequencing have elucidated the genetics of low-grade glioma. Available evidence indicates a neomorphic mutation in isocitrate dehydrogenase (IDH) initiates gliomagenesis. Mutant IDH produces the oncometabolite 2-hydroxyglutarate, which inhibits enzymes that demethylate genomic DNA and histones. Recent findings by the authors and others suggest the ensuing hypermethylation alters chromatin conformation and the transcription factor landscape in brain progenitor cells, leading to a block in differentiation and tumor initiation. Work in preclinical models has identified selective metabolic and molecular vulnerabilities of low-grade glioma. These new concepts will trigger a wave of innovative clinical trials in the near future.

Glioma cells diffusely infiltrate the surrounding brain tissue where they intermingle with nonneoplastic brain cells, including astrocytes, microglia, oligodendrocytes and neurons. The infiltrative margins of glioma represent the structural and functional interface between neoplastic and nonneoplastic brain tissue that underlies neurologic alterations associated with glioma, including epilepsy and neurologic deficits. Technological advancements in molecular analysis, including single cell sequencing, now allow us to assess alterations in specific cell types in the brain tumor microenvironment, which can enhance the development of novel therapies that target glioma growth and glioma-induced neurologic symptoms.

Clinical and Imaging

Clinical Presentation, Natural History, and Prognosis of Diffuse Low-Grade Gliomas   35

Anja Smits and Asgeir S. Jakola

Diffuse low-grade gliomas (DLGGs) are primary brain tumors characterized by slow growth but extensive infiltration into the surrounding brain. Patients are typically 30 to 40 years at disease onset and present with focal or focal to bilateral tonic-clonic seizures. The tumor will transform into a malignant glioma and eventually lead to death, but after varying lengths of time. The specific features of DLGG impose a major challenge to decide optimal treatment strategies and timing of treatment, while maintaining patients' quality of life. We discuss the clinical challenges at disease onset with regard to the natural history and long-term prognosis.

Diffuse Low-Grade Glioma-Related Epilepsy   43

Johan Pallud and Guy M. McKhann

The World Health Organization classifies diffuse low-grade gliomas (DLGGs) are highly epileptogenic primary brain tumors; epileptic seizures occur in more than 90% of cases. Epileptic seizures and drug resistance progress during the course of DLGGs. The glioma-related epileptogenic mechanisms are multifactorial; epileptogenic foci lie within the infiltrated peritumoral neocortex. A short seizure duration before surgery and a large extent of resection are the main predictors of postoperative seizure control in DLGGs. A supratotal resection of a DLGG can improve postoperative seizure control. Epileptic seizure at diagnosis positively affects DLGGs malignant transformation and overall survival.

Treatment

Mapping in Low-Grade Glioma Surgery: Low- and High-Frequency Stimulation   55

Marco Rossi, Sepehr Sani, Marco Conti Nibali, Luca Fornia, Lorenzo Bello, and Richard W. Byrne

Surgery for lower grade glioma requires the use of brain mapping techniques to identify functional boundaries, which represent the limit of the resection. Two stimulation paradigms are currently available and their use should be tailored to the clinical context to extend tumor removal and decrease the odds of postoperative permanent deficits.

Surgical Adjuncts to Increase the Extent of Resection: Intraoperative MRI, Fluorescence, and Raman Histology   65

Todd Hollon, Walter Stummer, Daniel Orringer, and Eric Suero Molina

In low-grade glioma surgery, depicting tumor margins is challenging. Several tools have emerged to assist surgical decision-making. Intraoperative MRI, albeit expensive and time-consuming, can provide useful information during surgery. Fluorescence-guidance with 5-aminolevulinic acid (5-ALA) helps provide real-time information during surgery regardless of brain-shift, assists in finding anaplastic foci in low-grade tumors, and enables diagnosis of malignant tissue. Raman histology has potential for detecting viable tumor in biopsied tissue and for identifying tumor infiltration in vivo. This article analyzes and discusses these surgical adjuncts.

Low-grade gliomas represent an important class of primary brain tumors. They account for approximately 20% of primary brain tumors and typically present in the fourth decade of life. Standard management gliomas involves observation, surgery, chemotherapy, and/or radiotherapy. Treatment decisions are based on many factors including prognostic molecular markers, potential benefits of increased progression-free survival, and potential long-term treatment complications. Recent studies have improved our understanding regarding therapeutic interventions. This review provides an overview of low-grade glioma and discusses the roles of radiation therapy. We discuss advances in techniques and recent and ongoing radiation therapy-related clinical trials for low-grade gliomas.

Diffuse low-grade glioma (DLGG) is a brain neoplasm that migrates within the connectome and that becomes malignant if left untreated. Early and maximal safe surgical resection by means of awake mapping enables a significant improvement of survival and quality of life. Supramaximal functional-based resection seems to prevent DLGG malignant transformation. Neuroplasticity is helpful to remove DLGG in eloquent areas. When radical excision cannot be achieved due to invasion of critical neural networks, cerebral remapping over time may lead to a reoperation with an optimized resection. To discover and treat DLGG earlier, a screening in the general population should be considered.

For the neurosurgical oncologist, a specialty practice in gliomas represents an intersection of tailored surgical approaches, emerging intraoperative technologies, expanding surgical trial portfolios, and new paradigms in glioma biology. Assembling these disparate pieces into a cohesive career trajectory is a difficult task but ultimately enables the subspecialist to navigate all domains relevant to improving glioma patient outcomes. Within the larger clinical and basic science community, thoughtful integration and intensive collaborations are essential mechanisms when building a multidisciplinary glioma program.

NEUROSURGERY CLINICS OF NORTH AMERICA

SERIES OF RELATED INTEREST

Neurologic Clinics
http://www.neurologicclinics.com
Neuroimaging Clinics
http://www.neuroimaging.theclinics.com/

THE CLINICS ARE AVAILABLE ONLINE!
Access your subscription at:
www.theclinics.com

NEUROSURGERY CLINICS OF NORTH AMERICA

FORTHCOMING ISSUES

April 2019
Neuromodulation
Wendell Lake, Ashwini Sharan, and
Chengyuan Wu, Editors

July 2019
Lumbar Spondylolisthesis
Zaher Ghogawala, Editor

October 2019
Pituitary Adenoma
Manish K. Aghi and Lewis S. Blevins, Editors

RECENT ISSUES

October 2018
Coagulation and Hematology in Neurological Surgery
Shahid M. Nimjee and Russell R. Lonser, Editors

July 2018
Degenerative Spinal Deformity: Creating Lordosis in the Lumbar Spine
Sigurd Berven and Praveen V. Mummaneni, Editors

April 2018
Neurocritical Care
Alejandro A. Rabinstein, Editor

SERIES OF RELATED INTEREST

Neurologic Clinics
http://www.neurologic.theclinics.com
Neuroimaging Clinics
http://www.neuroimaging.theclinics.com/

Preface

Low-Grade Glioma: Epidemiology, Pathophysiology, Clinical Features, and Treatment

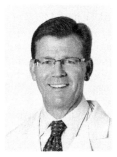   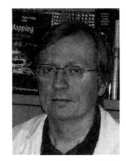

Guy M. McKhann, MD   Hugues Duffau, MD, PhD

Editors

The treatment of low-grade gliomas (LGGs) continues to evolve and improve as the field of Neurosurgery incorporates progressive advances in neuroimaging, molecular and cellular pathophysiology, extraoperative and intraoperative brain mapping, intraoperative surgical adjuncts, and postsurgical treatment with radiation and chemotherapy. While as surgeons we focus primarily on the surgical treatment of LGG patients, in order to provide optimal care for our patients we need to understand all aspects of their disease process. In this issue of *Neurosurgery Clinics of North America*, we have assembled an international panel of experts in the LGG field to discuss the latest advances in our understanding of the epidemiology, pathophysiology, clinical aspects, and treatment of these complex tumors.

The initial articles in this issue overview the epidemiology, classification, and molecular pathogenesis of LGGs. The WHO classification (2016) of LGGs stratifies these tumors based upon mutations in isocitrate dehydrogenase (IDH) and co-deletion of chromosomes 1p and 19q into separate diagnostic and prognostic groups. IDH–wild-type astrocytomas are the most aggressive LGGs, while IDH mutant, P53/ATRX mutated astrocytic LGGs have an intermediate prognosis, and IDH mutant, 1p/19q co-deleted oligodendrogliomas generally have a less aggressive clinical course. Studying the molecular pathophysiology of LGG has provided fundamental insights into gliomagenesis and provided potential opportunities to target novel treatments to these tumors.

The pathology, clinical course, and in particular epileptogenesis seen in LGG patients depends in large part upon the many ways that these tumors invade and interact with surrounding brain tissue. These issues are examined in depth in the articles of this issue. While the possible malignant progression that occurs in LGG patients appropriately remains at the forefront of clinical care, the day-to-day quality of life experienced by our patients is in large part determined by tumor cell interactions with local neuronal, glial, and blood-brain barrier elements. These areas of brain pathophysiology and patient care will require much further study going forward.

The majority of this issue focuses on aspects of treatment of LGG patients. Several articles detail important surgical considerations, in particular, ways to increase the extent of resection of these

Neurosurg Clin N Am 30 (2019) xiii–xiv
https://doi.org/10.1016/j.nec.2018.10.001
1042-3680/19/© 2018 Published by Elsevier Inc.

infiltrating brain tumors. Specific topics include when and how to use low- versus high-frequency stimulation for intraoperative mapping of LGG patients; intraoperative surgical adjuncts to increase extent of resection, including intraoperative MRI, fluorescence imaging, and Raman spectroscopy; mapping "higher" brain functions, including cognition and emotion; and the evidence that greater extent of resection improves patient outcome. Articles on chemotherapy and radiation therapy for LGG summarize the latest trials in these areas. The remaining articles tackle a variety of topics of importance to neurosurgeons: how the impact of extent of resection is altered by molecular classification in LGG; supramaximal resection, neuroplasticity, and LGG screening; and the fundamentals of building a glioma clinical practice.

To care for LGG patients and advance the field further requires a multidisciplinary team of experts specializing in neuro-oncology, epilepsy neurology, neurosurgery, neuropathology, neuroradiology, neurophysiology, molecular and cellular neuroscience, neuropsychology, and rehabilitation. This issue of *Neurosurgery Clinics of North America* strives to update the latest information on LGG in the majority of these interrelated disciplines.

Guy M. McKhann, MD
Department of Neurological Surgery
Columbia University Medical Center/
New York Presbyterian Hospital
Neurological Institute
Room 411, 710 West 168th Street
New York, NY 10032, USA

Hugues Duffau, MD, PhD
Department of Neurosurgery
Gui de Chauliac Hospital
Montpellier University Medical Center
80, Avenue Augustin Fliche
Montpellier 34295, France

Institute for Neuroscience of Montpellier
INSERM U1051
Saint Eloi Hospital
Montpellier University Medical Center
Montpellier, France

E-mail addresses:
gm317@columbia.edu (G.M. McKhann)
h-duffau@chu-montpellier.f (H. Duffau)

Epidemiology, Pathophysiology, and Classification

Epidemiology and Molecular Epidemiology

Luc Bauchet, MD, PhD[a], Quinn T. Ostrom, PhD, MPH[b],*

KEYWORDS

- Low-grade glioma • Diffuse glioma • Epidemiology • Incidence • Survival • Population-based

KEY POINTS

- The recent revision of the WHO classification of CNS tumors and the new epidemiologic data underscore the link between diffuse low-grade gliomas (DLGG) and diffuse anaplastic gliomas (DAG). DLGG and DAG include grade II and grade III astrocytomas and oligodendrogliomas, and represent 22.6% of all glioma diagnosed in the United States. The most common histology is diffuse astrocytoma.
- Overall incidence of DLGG and DAG in the United States is 1.23 per 100,000; however, incidence varies by histologic type of tumor, age at diagnosis, sex, and race/ethnicity.
- Numerous factors have been shown to be associated with DLGG and DAG prognosis, including age, sex, extent of resection, and molecular characteristics.
- Many environmental and genetic risk factors have been studied for glioma; consistent evidence has been found for ionizing radiation exposure (which increases risk), allergies (which decreases risk), and for alleles at a specific set of 18 single-nucleotide polymorphisms (which increase risk).

INTRODUCTION

Gliomas represent approximately one-third of all primary brain and central nervous system (CNS) tumors diagnosed in the Western world, and approximately 80% of malignant primary brain and CNS tumors.[1–3] These tumors are classified using World Health Organization (WHO) grade criteria (I to IV), and are classified into multiple specific histologic subtypes, based on apparent cell type of origin and molecular characteristics.[4] According to the 2007 WHO classification of CNS tumors,[5] diffuse low-grade gliomas (DLGGs) are infiltrative WHO grade II glioma and include diffuse astrocytomas (fibrillary astrocytoma, gemistocytic astrocytoma, protoplasmic astrocytoma), oligodendroglioma, and oligoastrocytoma. The 2016 WHO classification[4] presents major restructuring of diffuse gliomas, including the following:

1. Uses molecular parameters to define many tumor entities, including mutations in isocitrate dehydrogenase 1/2 (*IDH1/2*), and deletion of the p arm of chromosome 1 and q arm of chromosome 19.
2. Several histologies have been removed, including fibrillary astrocytoma and protoplasmic astrocytoma.
3. The diagnosis of oligoastrocytoma/anaplastic oligoastrocytoma is strongly discouraged.

This revision also underscores the link between DLGG and diffuse anaplastic gliomas (DAG; including anaplastic astrocytoma and anaplastic

Disclosure Statement: Dr. Ostrom supported by a Research Training Grant from the Cancer Prevention and Research Institute of Texas (CPRIT; RP160097T).
[a] Department of Neurosurgery, Montpellier University Medical Center, National Institute for Health and Medical Research (INSERM), U1051, Hôpital Gui de Chauliac, Centre Hospitalo-Universitaire, 80 Avenue Augustin Fliche, Montpellier, France; [b] Department of Medicine, Section of Epidemiology and Population Sciences, Dan Duncan Comprehensive Cancer Center, Baylor College of Medicine, One Baylor Plaza, Houston, TX 77030-3498, USA
* Corresponding author.
E-mail address: Quinn.ostrom@bcm.edu

Table 1
Counts, annual age-adjusted incidence rates, and 95% confidence intervals for selected diffuse WHO grade II and grade III glioma histologies in the United States, 2010–2014

	Diffuse Astrocytoma			Anaplastic Astrocytoma			Oligodendroglioma			Anaplastic Oligodendroglioma		
	Count	AAAIR[a]	95% CI	Count	AAAIR[a]	95% CI	Count	AAAIR[a]	95% CI	Count	AAAIR[a]	95% CI
Overall	7793	0.48	0.47–0.49	6537	0.40	0.39–0.41	3753	0.24	0.23–0.25	1718	0.11	0.10–0.11
Sex												
Males	4314	0.55	0.54–0.57	3534	0.46	0.44–0.47	2105	0.28	0.26–0.29	966	0.12	0.11–0.13
Females	3479	0.42	0.41–0.43	2953	0.35	0.33–0.36	1648	0.21	0.20–0.22	752	0.09	0.09–0.10
Age												
0–14	768	0.25	0.23–0.27	294	0.10	0.09–0.11	110	0.04	0.03–0.04	—[b]	—[b]	—[b]
0–4	284	0.28	0.25–0.32	75	0.08	0.06–0.09	18	0.02	0.01–0.03	—[b]	—[b]	—[b]
5–9	224	0.22	0.19–0.25	103	0.11	0.09–0.13	40	0.04	0.03–0.20	—[b]	—[b]	—[b]
10–14	260	0.25	0.22–0.28	111	0.11	0.09–0.13	52	0.05	0.04–0.07	—[b]	—[b]	—[b]
15–39+	2283	0.44	0.42–0.46	1552	0.30	0.29–0.32	1440	0.28	0.27–0.30	439	0.09	0.08–0.10
40+	4742	0.64	0.62–0.66	4691	0.63	0.61–0.65	2203	0.31	0.30–0.32	1269	0.17	0.16–0.18
Race												
White	6829	0.53	0.51–0.54	5817	0.44	0.43–0.45	3308	0.27	0.26–0.28	1512	0.12	0.11–0.12
Black	596	0.29	0.26–0.31	423	0.21	0.19–0.23	229	0.11	0.10–0.13	94	0.05	0.04–0.06
AIAN	58	0.28	0.21–0.37	43	0.21	0.15–0.29	30	0.13	0.09–0.19	—[b]	—[b]	—[b]
API	253	0.28	0.25–0.32	205	0.23	0.20–0.27	147	0.16	0.13–0.19	91	0.10	0.08–0.12

Abbreviations: AAAIR, annual age-adjusted incidence rates; AIAN, American Indian/Alaska Native; API, Asian Pacific Islander; CI, confidence interval.

[a] All rates adjusted to the US 2000 Census population.

[b] Counts and rates are not presented when fewer than 16 cases were reported.

Data from Ostrom QT, Gittleman H, Liao P, et al. CBTRUS statistical report: primary brain and other central nervous system tumors diagnosed in the United States in 2010 to 2014. Neuro Oncol 2017;19(suppl_5):v1–88.

oligodendroglioma). It is not currently known if DAG (WHO grade III) arise from initially DLGG (WHO grade II), or if these represent a separate entity. The resolution of this question is important to glioma epidemiology, because it may change the way these tumors are classified, and therefore patterns of incidence and prevalence. More information on the classification of these tumors is discussed in Devin Bready and Dimitris G. Placantonakis' article, "Molecular Pathogenesis of Low-Grade Glioma," in this issue.

The 2016 WHO Classification is new, and as a result, no population-level data using this scheme are available in brain tumor registries. Only specific studies that include molecular parameters are available. In this article, we only describe epidemiology for DLGG defined by the previous WHO classification (based on histology), and give some complementary data for DAG.

INCIDENCE

The overall age-adjusted incidence rate of DLGG and DAG (including WHO grade II and WHO grade III astrocytomas and oligodendrogliomas) was 1.23 per 100,000 population in the United States between 2010 and 2014. These tumors represent 22.6% of all gliomas diagnosed in the United States.[1] The most commonly diagnosed type of DLGG and DAG is diffuse astrocytoma (**Table 1**). Because of the relatively recent adoption of molecular markers in the classification of these tumors, all population-based estimates are based on histologic definitions.

Incidence by Sex

These tumors are more common in males, who have approximately 30% higher incidence as compared with females. Incidence by sex is shown by selected glioma histologies in **Table 1**.

Incidence by Age

The patterns of incidence for each histology vary by age. Median age at diagnosis is younger for DLGG and higher for DAG.[1,2] Incidence by age is shown by selected glioma histologies in **Fig. 1** and **Table 1**.

Incidence by Race

Incidence of glioma is highest among white persons and individuals of European descent. Incidence by race in the United States is shown by selected glioma histologies in **Table 1**. As compared with white persons, incidence of DLGG is approximately 45% lower in all other racial groups.

Global Incidence

Incidence of glioma varies significantly by region of the globe. Country- and region-specific rates are shown by selected glioma histologies in **Table 2**. Overall, global incidence of astrocytic tumors is highest (2.98/100,000 person-years), followed by oligodendroglial tumors (0.43/100,000 person-years).

Incidence Time Trends

Time trends in cancer incidence rates are an important measure of the changing burden of cancer in a population over time. Many things can affect incidence rates, including demographic changes, changes in histologic classification, and changes in cancer registration procedures. Recent changes in glioma incidence have been small. In the United States and in other more developed countries, incidence has been steady in adults, whereas incidence in children has been increasing slightly.[1,6]

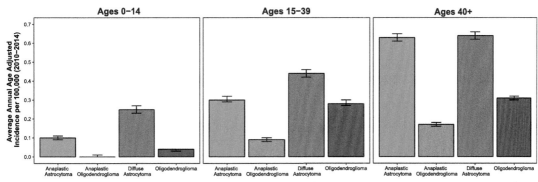

Fig. 1. Average annual incidence rates per 100,000 population of selected diffuse WHO grade II and grade III glioma histologies in the United States by age at diagnosis. (*Data from* Ostrom QT, Gittleman H, Liao P, et al. CBTRUS statistical report: primary brain and other central nervous system tumors diagnosed in the United States in 2010–2014. Neuro Oncol 2017;19(suppl_5):v1–88.)

Table 2
Age-adjusted incidence rates/100,000 persons for selected diffuse WHO grade II and grade III glioma histologies, by country/region and gender (all ages)

Histologic Type	Region (Organization)	Years	Rate[a]	95% CI
Diffuse astrocytoma ICD-O-3 morphology codes 9400, 9410–9411, 9420	The Netherlands[59]	1989–2010	0.50[b]	
	United States[1] (CBTRUS)	2010–2014	0.48[c]	0.47–0.49
	France (FBTDB)[2]	2006–2011	0.15[b]	
Anaplastic astrocytoma ICD-O-3 morphology code 9401	Austria[3] (ABTR)	2005	0.44[c]	0.33–0.58
	Korea[60]	2005	0.13	
	The Netherlands[59]	1989–2010	0.60[b]	
	United States[1] (CBTRUS)	2010–2014	0.40[c]	0.39–0.41
	France[2] (FBTDB)	2006–2011	0.16[b]	
Oligodendroglioma ICD-O-3 morphology code 9450	Austria[3] (ABTR)	2005	0.20[c]	0.13–0.30
	England[58]	1999–2003	0.21	
	Korea[60]	2005	0.10	
	The Netherlands[59]	1989–2010	0.20[b]	
	United States[1] (CBTRUS)	2010–2014	0.24[c]	0.23–0.25
	France[2] (FBTDB)	2006–2011	0.50[b]	
Anaplastic oligodendroglioma ICD-O-3 morphology codes 9451, 9460	Korea[60]	2005	0.06	
	The Netherlands[59]	1989–2010	0.20[b]	
	United States[1] (CBTRUS)	2010–2014	0.11[c]	0.10–0.11
	France[2] (FBTDB)	2006–2011	0.39[b]	
Astrocytic tumors (includes WHO grade IV glioblastoma) ICD-O-3 morphology codes 9384, 9400–9421, 9424, 9440–9442	Global[61]	2003–2007	2.98	2.97–3.00
	Australia and New Zealand[61]	2003–2007	3.94	3.83–4.05
	Canada[61]	2003–2007	3.58	3.49–3.67
	East Asia[61]	2003–2007	0.96	0.93–0.99
	Eastern Europe and Central Asia[61]	2003–2007	2.21	2.17–2.25
	India[61]	2003–2007	1.50	1.45–1.56
	Latin America[61]	2003–2007	2.09	2.01–2.16
	Middle East and North Africa[61]	2003–2007	2.39	2.31–2.48
	Northern Europe[61]	2003–2007	2.98	2.94–3.03
	Southeast Asia[61]	2003–2007	0.93	0.87–0.99
	Southeast Africa[61]	2003–2007	0.13	0.07–0.21
	Southern Europe[61]	2003–2007	3.01	2.95–3.08
	United States[61]	2003–2007	3.59	3.56–3.62
	Western Europe[61]	2003–2007	3.59	3.53–3.65
Oligodendroglial tumors and mixed glioma ICD-O-3 morphology codes 9382, 9450–9451	Global[61]	2003–2007	0.43	0.42–0.43
	Australia and New Zealand[61]	2003–2007	0.64	0.6–0.69
	Canada[61]	2003–2007	0.67	0.64–0.71
	East Asia[61]	2003–2007	0.20	0.19–0.21
	Eastern Europe and Central Asia[61]	2003–2007	0.26	0.25–0.28
	India[61]	2003–2007	0.18	0.16–0.2
	Latin America[61]	2003–2007	0.29	0.27–0.32
	Middle East and North Africa[61]	2003–2007	0.31	0.28–0.34
	Northern Europe[61]	2003–2007	0.45	0.44–0.47
	Southeast Asia[61]	2003–2007	0.11	0.09–0.14
	Southeast Africa[61]	2003–2007	—	—
	Southern Europe[61]	2003–2007	0.37	0.34–0.39
	United States[61]	2003–2007	0.56	0.55–0.57
	Western Europe[61]	2003–2007	0.61	0.59–0.64

Abbreviations: ABTR, Austrian Brain Tumor Registry; CBTRUS, Central Brain Tumor Registry of the United States; CI, confidence interval; FBTDB, French Brain Tumor Database; ICD, International Classification of Diseases.
[a] Rate in person-years, adjusted to the WHO standard population unless otherwise stated.
[b] Adjusted to the European standard population.
[c] Adjusted to the US 2000 Census population.
Data from Refs.[1–3,58–61]

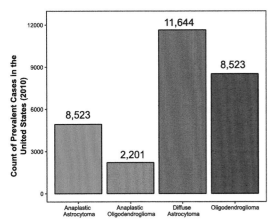

Fig. 2. Estimated count of prevalent cases for selected diffuse WHO grade II and grade III glioma histologies in the United States in 2010. (*Data from* Zhang AS, Ostrom QT, Kruchko C, et al. Complete prevalence of malignant primary brain tumors registry data in the United States compared with other common cancers, 2010. Neuro Oncol 2017;19(5):726–35.)

PREVALENCE

Prevalence is the estimate of the total number of individuals with a disease alive within a population, as compared with incidence, which counts new diagnoses only. It was estimated that there were 147,219 prevalent cases of primary malignant brain tumors in the United States in 2010, of which 21.3% are DLGG or DAG.[7] The prevalence of these tumors is more than 50% higher than glioblastoma (GBM, WHO grade IV astrocytoma), even though GBM represents most glioma diagnoses.[7,8] Estimated prevalent cases are shown by selected histologies in **Figs. 2** and **3**.

SURVIVAL

Relative survival (RS) after diagnosis with glioma varies significant by histology, with the best survival outcomes in oligodendroglioma. RS rates by selected histologies are shown in **Fig. 4**.

Survival by Age

RS after diagnosis with glioma varies significantly by age. In general, survival is highest in younger age groups. RS rates by selected histologies and age in the United States are shown in **Fig. 5**.

Global Survival

Survival after diagnosis with a DLGG or DAG varies significantly across the globe. In general, survival is highest in the United States. RS rates are listed by country and selected histologies in **Table 3**.

PROGNOSTIC FACTORS AND CLINICAL EPIDEMIOLOGY

Clinical epidemiology researchers have identified many prognostic factors for DLGG. **Table 4** provides a summary of these factors, and discussion elsewhere.[8,9] These data are not often collected at a population level, and most research is based on single-institution or clinical trials datasets. The developments of modern informatics technology have revolutionized data collection methods, and now allow for recording of all patient characteristics, treatment patterns, and outcomes. It may soon be possible to determine the best therapeutic sequences at the individual level based on identified prognostic factors. It is difficult to conduct large clinical trials in DLGG, because of their rarity, long survival, and brain plasticity. The development of dedicated databases is also crucial for recording treatment side effects and analyzing the quality of life.

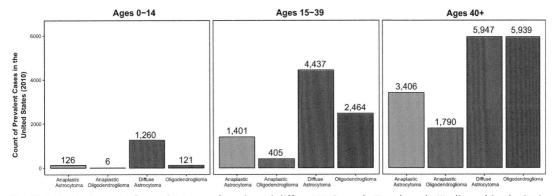

Fig. 3. Estimated count of prevalent cases for selected diffuse WHO grade II and grade III glioma histologies in the United States in 2010 by age at prevalence. (*Data from* Zhang AS, Ostrom QT, Kruchko C, et al. Complete prevalence of malignant primary brain tumors registry data in the United States compared with other common cancers, 2010. Neuro Oncol 2017;19(5):726–35.)

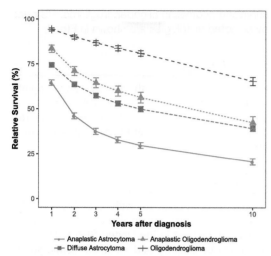

Fig. 4. The 1-, 2-, 3-, 4-, 5-, and 10-year relative survival after diagnosis with selected diffuse WHO grade II and grade III glioma histologies in the United States. (*Data from* Ostrom QT, Gittleman H, Liao P, et al. CBTRUS statistical report: primary brain and other central nervous system tumors diagnosed in the United States in 2010–2014. Neuro Oncol 2017;19(suppl_5):v1–88.)

ENVIRONMENTAL RISK FACTORS
Allergies

Allergies have been reported to be protective against multiple cancer types, including all glioma, where a recent meta-analysis estimated that allergies reduce overall glioma risk by nearly 40%.[10,11] Studies have consistently shown that history of atopic conditions (including asthma, hay fever, eczema, and food allergies) lead to reduced glioma risk (see **Fig. 6**A for a summary of studies[10,12–15]). Several potential mechanisms

for this protective effect have been proposed, including: increased surveillance by the innate immune system, similarity between antibodies and brain tumor antigens, or increased effectiveness of response to environmental carcinogens.[16,17]

Ionizing Radiation

Multiple studies have evaluated the association between even low doses of therapeutic radiation and brain tumors (see **Fig. 6**B for a summary of studies[18–22]). Low doses of therapeutic radiation have been shown to increase risk for all glioma three-fold,[20] and there is increased risk of brain tumors in individuals with prior radiation treatment of cancer.[18,21,22] The effect of diagnostic radiation exposures (eg, computed tomography scans or MRIs) on the development of brain tumors remains unclear.[23]

Cellular Phones

After its introduction in the 1980s, cellular telephone technology is now ubiquitous. This has led to public concern over the potential disease risk related to the nonionizing radiation emitted by cellular phones (see **Fig. 6**C for a summary of recent studies[24–26]). In 2011, the International Agency for Research on Cancer found that radiation produced by cellular phones is a possible carcinogen,[27] based largely on findings for self-reported heavy users. A separate review concluded that research did not support a relationship between cellular phone use and all glioma.[28] Multiple additional studies have further explored this relationship. Two cohort studies using subscription records found no increase in all glioma,[24,25] whereas several case-control studies

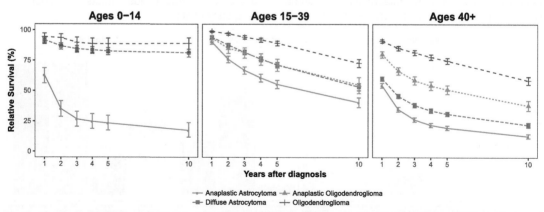

Fig. 5. The 1-, 2-, 3-, 4-, 5-, and 10-year relative survival after diagnosis with selected diffuse WHO grade II and grade III glioma histologies in the United States by age. (*Data from* Ostrom QT, Gittleman H, Liao P, et al. CBTRUS statistical report: primary brain and other central nervous system tumors diagnosed in the United States in 2010–2014. Neuro Oncol 2017;19(suppl_5):v1–88.)

Table 3
Relative survival for selected diffuse WHO grade II and grade III glioma histologies and country/region (all ages)

Histologic Type	Region (Organization)	Years	1-y (95% CI)	5-y (95% CI)	10-y (95% CI)
Diffuse astrocytoma ICD-O-3 morphology codes 9400, 9410–9411, 9420	United States[1] (CBTRUS)	2000–2014	74.7 (73.5–75.8)	50.1 (48.7–51.5)	39.3 (37.8–40.9)
Anaplastic astrocytoma ICD-O-3 morphology code 9401	Korea[63]	1994–2004	64.3	25.2	
	Taiwan[62]	2002–2010	67.8 (63.2–71.9)	22.1 (18.1–26.3)	
	United Kingdom and Ireland[64] (EUROCARE)	1995–2002		17.6 (13.5–22.2)	
	Northern Europe[64] (EUROCARE)	1995–2002		10.8 (7.8–14.4)	
	Central Europe[64] (EUROCARE)	1995–2002		28.8 (19.3–39.0)	
	Eastern Europe[64] (EUROCARE)	1995–2002		11.7 (7.1–17.4)	
	Southern Europe[64] (EUROCARE)	1995–2002		18.1 (11.8–25.4)	
	United States[1] (CBTRUS)	2000–2014	64.9 (63.3–66.3)	29.8 (28.2–31.4)	20.8 (19.1–22.5)
Oligodendroglioma ICD-O-3 morphology code 9450	Korea[63]	1994–2004	77.3	73.5	
	Taiwan[62]	2002–2010	91.9 (88.0–94.5)	70.3 (64.5–75.4)	
	United Kingdom and Ireland[64] (EUROCARE)	1995–2002		65.8 (57.5–73.0)	
	Northern Europe[64] (EUROCARE)	1995–2002		74.1 (64.4–81.8)	
	Central Europe[64] (EUROCARE)	1995–2002		75.5 (61.8–85.2)	
	Eastern Europe[64] (EUROCARE)	1995–2002		47.8 (32.4–62.0)	
	Southern Europe[64] (EUROCARE)	1995–2002		63.8 (51.4–74.1)	
	United States[1] (CBTRUS)	2000–2014	94.5 (93.6–95.3)	81.3 (79.7–82.8)	65.7 (63.4–67.9)
Anaplastic oligodendroglioma ICD-O-3 morphology codes 9451, 9460	Korea[63]	1994–2004	84.5	50.4	
	Taiwan[62]	2002–2010	82.7 (75.6–87.9)	35.4 (27.3–43.7)	
	United Kingdom and Ireland[64] (EUROCARE)	1995–2002		35.5 (24.4–46.9)	
	Northern Europe[64] (EUROCARE)	1995–2002		35.1 (21.2–49.5)	
	Central Europe[64] (EUROCARE)	1995–2002		29.7 (13.4–48.3)	
	Eastern Europe[64] (EUROCARE)	1995–2002		6.1 (1.3–16.6)	
	Southern Europe[64] (EUROCARE)	1995–2002		33.3 (14.7–53.6)	
	United States[1] (CBTRUS)	2000–2014	83.9 (81.7–85.8)	56.6 (53.6–59.5)	42.6 (39.1–46.0)
Oligodendroglial tumors ICD-O-3 morphology codes 9450–9451, 9460 and site codes C71, C72.0, C72.8–C72.9	England and Wales[65]	1971–1995	75.9	39.6	19.9
	Europe[66] (RARECARE)	1995–2002	83.0	55.0	

Abbreviations: CBTRUS, Central Brain Tumor Registry of the United States; CI, confidence interval; EUROCARE, European Cancer Registry–based study on survival and care of patients with cancer; ICD, International Classification of Diseases; RARECARE, surveillance of rare cancer in Europe.
Data from Refs.[1,62–66]

Table 4
Main suspected/proposed prognostic factors for diffuse low-grade glioma

Factor	Favorable	Publication
Age	Younger age	Ostrom et al,[1] 2017
Sex	Female gender	Claus and Black,[67] 2006
Race	White race	Claus and Black,[67] 2006
Neurologic status	Absence of neurologic deficit	Pignatti et al,[68] 2002
Epilepsy	Presence of epilepsy associated with improved survival	Pallud et al,[69] 2014
Comorbidity	Absence of comorbidities may improve survival	General consideration, but no specific work for DLGG
KPS	High[a] KPS associated with improved survival	Chang et al,[70] 2009; Capelle et al,[71] 2013
Tumor location	Outside eloquent location	Chang et al,[70] 2009
Tumor volume	Smaller[a] tumors improve survival	Chang et al,[70] 2009 Capelle et al,[71] 2013
Tumor growth rate	Slower[a] growth improves survival	Pallud et al,[72] 2013
Histology	Oligodendroglioma	Ostrom et al,[1] 2017
Biology	*IDH1/2* mutation	Yan et al,[73] 2009
	Codeletion of chromosomes 1p and 19q	Hartmann et al,[74] 2011; Smith et al,[75] 2000
	Absence of *TP53* mutation	Okamoto et al,[76] 2004
Surgery	Resection vs watch-and-wait	Jakola et al,[77] 2012
	No residual volume or small[a] residual volume after resection	Sanai et al,[78] 2011; Duffau,[79] 2013
	Second surgery when feasible	Ramakrishna et al,[80] 2015
Chemotherapy (mainly PCV or TMZ) or/and radiotherapy	Many publications reported some benefit with chemotherapy and/or radiotherapy, particularly when complete resection is not feasible. There is no consensus about timing of these treatments, or which patients should receive these treatments	Buckner et al,[81] 2016; Weller et al,[82] 2017; Jhaveri et al,[83] 2018; Bady et al,[84] 2018; Mandonnet and Duffau,[85] 2018
Multistep therapeutic strategy	Likely improves survival, but needs further evaluation	Duffau and Taillandier,[86] 2015

Abbreviations: KPS, Karnofsky performance status; PCV, procarbazine, CCNU, and vincristine; IDH1/2: Isocitrate dehydrogenase 1/2; TMZ, temozolomide; TP53, tumor protein p53.
[a] See cutoff values in different publications.

using self-reported usage data have been published with mixed results.[26,29]

Although conflicted, the published studies do not demonstrate evidence of a significant association between cellular phone use and glioma. With increasing use earlier in life and the increased frequency of use, additional long-term studies are necessary to determine the true association between cellular phones and glioma.

Other Risk Factors

Many other potential risk factors have been explored, including: diet, viruses, reproductive factors, head injury, and exposure to electromagnetic fields. Associations between these factors and risk of brain and CNS tumor have not been

well replicated. A summary of investigated but unvalidated associations is listed next:

- Viruses, including simian virus 40, chicken pox, and cytomegalovirus[30–32]
- Occupational extremely low frequency electromagnetic field exposure[33]
- Exogenous hormonal drugs[34]
- Antihistamines[35,36]
- Nonsteroidal anti-inflammatory drugs[37]

HERITABLE GENETIC RISK FACTORS
Syndromic Brain Tumors

Several less common syndromes are also associated with the development of DLGG, DAG, or other brain tumors. **Table 5** provides an overview.

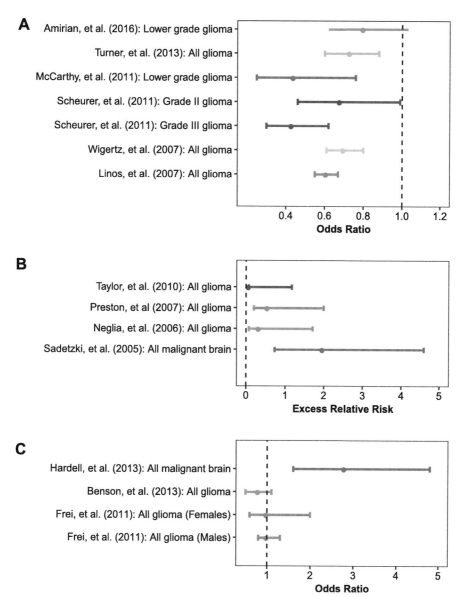

Fig. 6. Summary of recent studies of association between glioma and (A) history of allergy, (B) ionizing radiation exposure, and (C) cellular phone use. (*Data from* Refs.[10–15,17–24,88–91])

Familial Aggregation of Brain Tumors

Most cases of glioma are sporadic, meaning that they occur in individuals with no family history of these tumors. Approximately 5% are familial, meaning that a glioma has occurred multiple times within the same family.[38] There is approximately a two-fold to three-fold increase in risk of developing a brain tumor for first-degree relatives (parents, children, and full siblings) of individuals diagnosed with any glioma.[39–42] Risk of a glioma (including all grades) has also been found to also be elevated in individuals with family history of other cancers.[43]

Genetic studies have been conducted within affected glioma families (where more than one person has been diagnosed with a glioma of any grade) but have had little success identifying rare inherited genetic risk variants.[44,45] Additional analyses have found alterations in MutS protein homolog 2 (*MSH2*) and protection of telomeres 1 (*POT1*) that seem to be associated with glioma in a small number of families, but most mutations seem to be specific to each family.[46,47]

Genetic Risk Factors for Sporadic Glioma

Since advances in technology that now allow for rapid whole-genome genotyping, six genome-wide association studies of glioma patients have been conducted,[48–53] and have identified 18

Table 5
Inherited syndromes associated with glioma

Gene (Chromosome Location)	Disorder/Syndrome	Mode of Inheritance	Phenotypic Features	Associated Brain Tumors
NF1 (17q11.2)	Neurofibromatosis 1	Dominant	Neurofibromas, schwannomas, café-au-lait macules	Astrocytoma, optic nerve glioma
TSC1,TSC2 (9q34.14,16p13.3)	Tuberous sclerosis	Dominant	Development of multisystem nonmalignant tumors	Giant cell astrocytoma
MSH2,MLH1,MSH6,PMS2	Lynch syndrome	Dominant	Predisposition to gastrointestinal, endometrial, and other cancers	Glioblastoma, other gliomas
TP53 (17p13.1)	Li-Fraumeni syndrome	Dominant	Predisposition to numerous cancers, especially breast, brain, and soft tissue sarcoma	Glioblastoma, other gliomas
CDKN2A (9p21.3)	Melanoma-neural system tumor syndrome	Dominant	Predisposition to malignant melanoma and malignant brain tumors	Glioma
IDH1/IDH2 (2q33.3/15q26.1)	Ollier disease	Acquired post-zygotic mosaicism, dominant with reduced penetrance	Development of intraosseous benign cartilaginous tumors, cancer predisposition	Glioma
APC, MMR (5q21)	Turcot syndrome	Dominant	Development of multiple adenomatous colon polyps, predisposition to colorectal cancer, and brain tumors	Medulloblastoma, glioma
RB1 (13q14)	Retinoblastoma	Dominant	Development of multiple tumors of the eye, increased risk of some brain tumors	Retinoblastoma, pinealoblastoma, malignant glioma

Abbreviations: APC, adenomatous polyposis coli; CDKN2A, cyclin-dependent kinase Inhibitor 2A; IDH1, Isocitrate dehydrogenase 1; IDH2, Isocitrate dehydrogenase 2; MLH1, MutL homolog 1, colon cancer, nonpolyposis type 2; MSH2, MutS protein homolog 2; MSH6, MutS protein homolog 6; NF1, neurofibromin 1; NF2, neurofibromin 2; PMS2, PMS1 homolog 2, mismatch repair system component; PTCH1, patched 1; RB1, RB transcriptional corepressor 1; TP53, tumor protein p53; TSC1, TSC complex subunit 1; TSC2, TSC complex subunit 1; VHL, von Hippel-Lindau tumor suppressor.

Data from Farrell CJ, Plotkin SR. Genetic causes of brain tumors: neurofibromatosis, tuberous sclerosis, von Hippel-Lindau, and other syndromes. Neurol Clin 2007;25(4):925–46; and Melean G, Sestini R, Ammannati F, et al. Genetic insights into familial tumors of the nervous system. Am J Med Genet C Semin Med Genet 2004;129C(1):74–84.

Table 6
Heritable variants associated with diffuse WHO grade II and grade III risk from genome-wide association studies

Candidate Gene (Chromosome Location)	SNP-Risk Allele	Odds Ratio[a]	RAF in Europeans[b]	Associated Glioma Subtype	Studies Detected (y)
MDM4 (1q32.1)	rs4252707-A	1.19	0.220	Non-GBM glioma	Melin, et al,[48] 2017
AKT3 (1q44)	rs12076373-G	1.23	0.840	Non-GBM glioma	Melin et al,[48] 2017
C2orf80 (2q33.3)	rs7572263-A	1.20	0.760	Non-GBM glioma	Melin, et al,[48] 2017
LRIG1 (3p14.1)	rs11706832-C	1.15	0.460	Non-GBM glioma	Melin, et al,[48] 2017
TERT (5p15.33)	rs10069690-T	1.27	0.276	All glioma subtypes	Shete et al,[50] 2009; Wrensch, et al,[52] 2009; Sanson et al,[87] 2011; Rajamaran, et al,[51] 2012; Melin et al,[48] 2017
EGFR (7p11.2)	rs75061358-G	1.28	0.099	All glioma subtypes	Sanson et al,[87] 2011; Rajamaran, et al,[51] 2012; Walsh et al,[53] 2013; Melin et al,[48] 2017
CCDC26 (8q24.21)	rs55705857-G	3.39	0.05	Oligodendroglial tumors/ *IDH1/2*-mutant astrocytic tumors	Shete et al,[50] 2009; Jenkins et al,[54] 2012; Rajamaran et al,[51] 2012; Enciso-Mora et al,[88] 2013; Melin et al,[48] 2017
CDKN2B (9p21.3)	rs634537-G	1.21	0.410	Astrocytic tumors, WHO grades II-IV	Shete et al,[50] 2009; Wrensch et al,[52] 2009; Rajamaran et al,[51] 2012
STN1 (10q24.33)	rs11598018-C	1.14	0.462	Non-GBM glioma	Melin et al,[48] 2017
VTI1A (10q25.2)	rs11599775-G	1.16	0.620	Non-GBM glioma	Kinnersley et al,[49] 2015; Melin et al,[48] 2017

(continued on next page)

Table 6
(continued)

Candidate Gene (Chromosome Location)	SNP-Risk Allele	Odds Ratio[a]	RAF in Europeans[b]	Associated Glioma Subtype	Studies Detected (y)
MAML2 (11q21)	rs7107785-T	1.16	0.479	Non-GBM glioma	Melin et al,[48] 2017
PHLDB1 (11q23.2)	rs648044-A	1.42	0.390	Non-GBM glioma	Shete et al,[50] 2009; Melin et al,[48] 2017
PHLDB1 (11q23.3)	rs498872-A	1.50	0.320	IDH1/2-mutant gliomas	Shete et al,[50] 2009; Rajamaran et al,[51] 2012; Rice et al,[89] 2013
Intergenic (12q21.2)	rs1275600-T	1.16	0.595	Non-GBM glioma	Kinnersley et al,[49] 2015; Melin et al,[48] 2017
AKAP6 (14q12)	rs10131032-G	1.33	0.916	Non-GBM glioma	Melin et al,[48] 2017
ETFA (15q24.2)	rs1801591-A	1.35	0.086	Non-GBM glioma	Kinnersley et al,[49] 2015; Melin et al,[48] 2017
RHBDF1 (16p13.3)	rs3751667-T	1.18	0.208	Non-GBM glioma	Melin et al,[48] 2017
TP53 (17p13.1)	rs78378222-C	2.73	0.010	All glioma subtypes	Stacey et al,[90] 2011; Enciso-Mora et al,[91] 2013; Melin et al,[48] 2017
RTEL1 (20q13.33)	rs2297440-C	1.20	0.7960	All glioma subtypes	Shete et al,[50] 2009; Wrensch et al,[52] 2009; Rajamaran et al,[51] 2012; Melin et al,[48] 2017

Abbreviations: AKAP6, A-kinase anchoring protein 6'; AKT3, AKT serine/threonine kinase 3; C2orf80, chromosome 2 open reading frame 80; CCDC26, coiled-coil domain containing 26; CDKN2B, cyclin-dependent kinase inhibitor 2B; EGFR, epidermal growth factor receptor; ETFA, electron transfer flavoprotein alpha subunit; HEATR3, HEAT repeat containing 3; IDH1/2, Isocitrate dehydrogenase 1/2; LRG1, leucine rich repeats and immunoglobulin like domains 1; MAML2, mastermind like transcriptional coactivator 2; MDM4, MDM4, p53 regulator; PHLDB1, pleckstrin homology-like domain, family E, member 1; RHBDF1, rhomboid 5 homolog 1; RTEL1, regulator of telomere elongation helicase; SNP, single nucleotide polymorphism; STN1, STN1, CST complex subunit; TERT, telomerase reverse transcriptase; TP53, tumor protein p53; VTI1A, vesicle transport through interaction with t-SNAREs 1A.

  [a] Odds ratio estimates from Melin, et al. (2017)[48].

  [b] Allele frequencies within European super-population within the 1,000 genomes project.

Data from Melin BS, Barnholtz-Sloan JS, Wrensch MR, et al. Genome-wide association study of glioma subtypes identifies specific differences in genetic susceptibility to glioblastoma and non-glioblastoma tumors. Nat Genet 2017;49(5):789–94.

genomic variants (eg, single-nucleotide polymorphisms) that increased risk of non-GBM glioma (**Table 6**). Most analyses have used pooled samples of all non-GBM glioma subtypes, and have not explored specific molecular subtype associations. The identified variant near *CCDC26* has had the most extensive molecular subtype-specific exploration, and this single-nucleotide polymorphism is most strongly associated with oligodendroglial tumors with mutant *IDH1/2*, with no significant association for *IDH1/2* wild-type tumors.[54]

OTHER HYPOTHESIS FOR GLIOMA RISK

Beside epigenetic and gene-environment interaction that could be involved in the cause of many cancer, one specific other cause for glioma could be the functional theory. First, DLGG are preferentially located close (or in) functional areas.[55] Second, cerebral structural changes induced by training or specific activity have been reported in humans.[56] It is therefore possible to hypothesize that oversolicitation (or hyposolicitation) of functional networks by a specific task, association of task, or environmental demand, could favor.[8,57]

SUMMARY

Incidence, prevalence, and survival for DLGGs vary by histologic type, age at diagnosis, sex, and race/ethnicity. Significant progress has been made in identifying potential risk factors for gliomas, although more research is warranted. The strongest risk factors that have been identified thus far include allergies/atopic disease, ionizing radiation, and heritable genetic factors. Scientific evidence for an association between exposure to nonionizing radiation in the form of cellular phones and glioma risk is inconclusive. Modern clinical informatics systems and genome-wide "omic" technologies provide the opportunity to examine risk factors while accounting for the heterogeneity of these tumors.

REFERENCES

1. Ostrom QT, Gittleman H, Liao P, et al. CBTRUS statistical report: primary brain and other central nervous system tumors diagnosed in the United States in 2010-2014. Neuro Oncol 2017;19(suppl_5):v1–88.
2. Darlix A, Zouaoui S, Rigau V, et al. Epidemiology for primary brain tumors: a nationwide population-based study. J Neurooncol 2017;131(3):525–46.
3. Wohrer A, Waldhor T, Heinzl H, et al. The Austrian Brain Tumour Registry: a cooperative way to establish a population-based brain tumour registry. J Neurooncol 2009;95(3):401–11.
4. Louis DN, Perry A, Reifenberger G, et al. The 2016 World Health Organization classification of tumors of the central nervous system: a summary. Acta Neuropathol 2016;131(6):803–20.
5. Louis DN, Ohgaki H, Wiestler OD, et al. The 2007 WHO classification of tumours of the central nervous system. Acta Neuropathol 2007;114(2):97–109.
6. Gittleman HR, Ostrom QT, Rouse CD, et al. Trends in central nervous system tumor incidence relative to other common cancers in adults, adolescents, and children in the United States, 2000 to 2010. Cancer 2015;121(1):102–12.
7. Zhang AS, Ostrom QT, Kruchko C, et al. Complete prevalence of malignant primary brain tumors registry data in the United States compared with other common cancers, 2010. Neuro Oncol 2017;19(5):726–35.
8. Bauchet L. Epidemiology of diffuse low-grade gliomas. In: Duffau H, editor. Diffuse low-grade gliomas in adults. 2nd edition. London: Springer-Verlag; 2017. p. 9–30.
9. Jacobs DI, Claus EB, Wrensch MR. Molecular epidemiology of diffuse low-grade glioma. In: Duffau H, editor. Diffuse low-grade gliomas in adults. 2nd edition. London: Springer-Verlag; 2017. p. 55–72.
10. Amirian ES, Zhou R, Wrensch MR, et al. Approaching a scientific consensus on the association between allergies and glioma risk: a report from the glioma international case-control study. Cancer Epidemiol Biomarkers Prev 2016;25(2):282–90.
11. Turner MC, Krewski D, Armstrong BK, et al. Allergy and brain tumors in the INTERPHONE study: pooled results from Australia, Canada, France, Israel, and New Zealand. Cancer Causes Control 2013;24(5):949–60.
12. Linos E, Raine T, Alonso A, et al. Atopy and risk of brain tumors: a meta-analysis. J Natl Cancer Inst 2007;99(20):1544–50.
13. McCarthy BJ, Rankin K, Il'yasova D, et al. Assessment of type of allergy and antihistamine use in the development of glioma. Cancer Epidemiol Biomarkers Prev 2011;20(2):370–8.
14. Scheurer ME, Amirian ES, Davlin SL, et al. Effects of antihistamine and anti-inflammatory medication use on risk of specific glioma histologies. Int J Cancer 2011;129(9):2290–6.
15. Wigertz A, Lonn S, Schwartzbaum J, et al. Allergic conditions and brain tumor risk. Am J Epidemiol 2007;166(8):941–50.
16. Sherman PW, Holland E, Sherman JS. Allergies: their role in cancer prevention. Q Rev Biol 2008;83(4):339–62.
17. Jensen-Jarolim E, Achatz G, Turner MC, et al. AllergoOncology: the role of IgE-mediated allergy in cancer. Allergy 2008;63(10):1255–66.

18. Neglia JP, Robison LL, Stovall M, et al. New primary neoplasms of the central nervous system in survivors of childhood cancer: a report from the Childhood Cancer Survivor Study. J Natl Cancer Inst 2006;98(21):1528–37.

19. Preston DL, Ron E, Tokuoka S, et al. Solid cancer incidence in atomic bomb survivors: 1958-1998. Radiat Res 2007;168(1):1–64.

20. Sadetzki S, Chetrit A, Freedman L, et al. Long-term follow-up for brain tumor development after childhood exposure to ionizing radiation for tinea capitis. Radiat Res 2005;163(4):424–32.

21. Taylor AJ, Little MP, Winter DL, et al. Population-based risks of CNS tumors in survivors of childhood cancer: the British Childhood Cancer Survivor Study. J Clin Oncol 2010;28(36):5287–93.

22. Perkins SM, Dewees T, Shinohara ET, et al. Risk of subsequent malignancies in survivors of childhood leukemia. J Cancer Surviv 2013;7(4):544–50.

23. Davis F, Il'yasova D, Rankin K, et al. Medical diagnostic radiation exposures and risk of gliomas. Radiat Res 2011;175(6):790–6.

24. Benson VS, Pirie K, Schuz J, et al. Mobile phone use and risk of brain neoplasms and other cancers: prospective study. Int J Epidemiol 2013;42(3):792–802.

25. Frei P, Poulsen AH, Johansen C, et al. Use of mobile phones and risk of brain tumours: update of Danish cohort study. BMJ 2011;343:d6387.

26. Hardell L, Carlberg M, Soderqvist F, et al. Case-control study of the association between malignant brain tumours diagnosed between 2007 and 2009 and mobile and cordless phone use. Int J Oncol 2013;43(6):1833–45.

27. Baan R, Grosse Y, Lauby-Secretan B, et al. Carcinogenicity of radiofrequency electromagnetic fields. Lancet Oncol 2011;12(7):624–6.

28. Swerdlow AJ, Feychting M, Green AC, et al, International Commission for Non-Ionizing Radiation Protection Standing Committee on Epidemiology. Mobile phones, brain tumors, and the interphone study: where are we now? Environ Health Perspect 2011;119(11):1534–8.

29. Yoon S, Choi JW, Lee E, et al. Mobile phone use and risk of glioma: a case-control study in Korea for 2002-2007. Environ Health Toxicol 2015;30:e2015015.

30. Vilchez RA, Butel JS. SV40 in human brain cancers and non-Hodgkin's lymphoma. Oncogene 2003;22(33):5164–72.

31. Lee S-T, Bracci P, Zhou M, et al. Interaction of allergy history and antibodies to specific varicella zoster virus proteins on glioma risk. Int J Cancer 2014;134(9):2199–210.

32. Amirian ES, Marquez-Do D, Bondy ML, et al. Anti-human-cytomegalovirus immunoglobulin G levels in glioma risk and prognosis. Cancer Med 2013;2(1):57–62.

33. Koeman T, van den Brandt PA, Slottje P, et al. Occupational extremely low-frequency magnetic field exposure and selected cancer outcomes in a prospective Dutch cohort. Cancer Causes Control 2014;25:203–14.

34. Qi ZY, Shao C, Zhang X, et al. Exogenous and endogenous hormones in relation to glioma in women: a meta-analysis of 11 case-control studies. PLoS One 2013;8(7):e68695.

35. Scheurer ME, El-Zein R, Thompson PA, et al. Long-term anti-inflammatory and antihistamine medication use and adult glioma risk. Cancer Epidemiol Biomarkers Prev 2008;17(5):1277–81.

36. Amirian ES, Marquez-Do D, Bondy ML, et al. Antihistamine use and immunoglobulin E levels in glioma risk and prognosis. Cancer Epidemiol 2013;37(6):908–12.

37. Liu Y, Lu Y, Wang J, et al. Association between nonsteroidal anti-inflammatory drug use and brain tumour risk: a meta-analysis. Br J Clin Pharmacol 2014;78(1):58–68.

38. Wrensch M, Lee M, Miike R, et al. Familial and personal medical history of cancer and nervous system conditions among adults with glioma and controls. Am J Epidemiol 1997;145(7):581–93.

39. Malmer B, Henriksson R, Grönberg H. Familial brain tumours: genetics or environment? A nationwide cohort study of cancer risk in spouses and first-degree relatives of brain tumour patients. Int J Cancer 2003;106(2):260–3.

40. Malmer B, Grönberg H, Bergenheim AT, et al. Familial aggregation of astrocytoma in northern Sweden: an epidemiological cohort study. Int J Cancer 1999;81(3):366–70.

41. Hill DA, Inskip PD, Shapiro WR, et al. Cancer in first-degree relatives and risk of glioma in adults. Cancer Epidemiol Biomarkers Prev 2003;12(12):1443–8.

42. Scheurer ME, Etzel CJ, Liu M, et al. Aggregation of cancer in first-degree relatives of patients with glioma. Cancer Epidemiol Biomarkers Prev 2007;16(11):2491–5.

43. Scheurer ME, Etzel CJ, Liu M, et al. Familial aggregation of glioma: a pooled analysis. Am J Epidemiol 2010;172(10):1099–107.

44. Shete S, Lau CC, Houlston RS, et al. Genome-wide high-density SNP linkage search for glioma susceptibility loci: results from the Gliogene Consortium. Cancer Res 2011;71(24):7568–75.

45. Sun X, Vengoechea J, Elston R, et al. A variable age of onset segregation model for linkage analysis, with correction for ascertainment, applied to glioma. Cancer Epidemiol Biomarkers Prev 2012;21(12):2242–51.

46. Bainbridge MN, Armstrong GN, Gramatges MM, et al. Germline mutations in shelterin complex genes

are associated with familial glioma. J Natl Cancer Inst 2015;107(1):384.

47. Andersson U, Wibom C, Cederquist K, et al. Germline rearrangements in families with strong family history of glioma and malignant melanoma, colon, and breast cancer. Neuro Oncol 2014;16(10):1333–40.

48. Melin BS, Barnholtz-Sloan JS, Wrensch MR, et al. Genome-wide association study of glioma subtypes identifies specific differences in genetic susceptibility to glioblastoma and non-glioblastoma tumors. Nat Genet 2017;49(5):789–94.

49. Kinnersley B, Labussiere M, Holroyd A, et al. Genome-wide association study identifies multiple susceptibility loci for glioma. Nat Commun 2015;6:8559.

50. Shete S, Hosking FJ, Robertson LB, et al. Genome-wide association study identifies five susceptibility loci for glioma. Nat Genet 2009;41(8):899–904.

51. Rajaraman P, Melin BS, Wang Z, et al. Genome-wide association study of glioma and meta-analysis. Hum Genet 2012;131(12):1877–88.

52. Wrensch M, Jenkins RB, Chang JS, et al. Variants in the CDKN2B and RTEL1 regions are associated with high-grade glioma susceptibility. Nat Genet 2009;41(8):905–8.

53. Walsh KM, Anderson E, Hansen HM, et al. Analysis of 60 reported glioma risk SNPs replicates published GWAS findings but fails to replicate associations from published candidate-gene studies. Genet Epidemiol 2013;37(2):222–8.

54. Jenkins RB, Xiao Y, Sicotte H, et al. A low-frequency variant at 8q24.21 is strongly associated with risk of oligodendroglial tumors and astrocytomas with IDH1 or IDH2 mutation. Nat Genet 2012;44(10):1122–5.

55. Duffau H, Capelle L. Preferential brain locations of low-grade gliomas. Cancer 2004;100(12):2622–6.

56. Draganski B, Gaser C, Busch V, et al. Neuroplasticity: changes in grey matter induced by training. Nature 2004;427(6972):311–2.

57. Darlix A, Goze C, Rigau V, et al. The etiopathogenesis of diffuse low-grade gliomas. Crit Rev Oncol Hematol 2017;109:51–62.

58. Arora RS, Alston RD, Eden TO, et al. Are reported increases in incidence of primary CNS tumours real? An analysis of longitudinal trends in England, 1979-2003. Eur J Cancer 2010;46(9):1607–16.

59. Ho VK, Reijneveld JC, Enting RH, et al. Changing incidence and improved survival of gliomas. Eur J Cancer 2014;50(13):2309–18.

60. Lee CH, Jung KW, Yoo H, et al. Epidemiology of primary brain and central nervous system tumors in Korea. J Korean Neurosurg Soc 2010;48(2):145–52.

61. Leece R, Xu J, Ostrom QT, et al. Global incidence of malignant brain and other central nervous system tumors by histology, 2003-2007. Neuro Oncol 2017;19(11):1553–64.

62. Chien LN, Gittleman H, Ostrom QT, et al. Comparative brain and central nervous system tumor incidence and survival between the United States and Taiwan based on population-based registry. Front Public Health 2016;4:151.

63. Jung KW, Yoo H, Kong HJ, et al. Population-based survival data for brain tumors in Korea. J Neurooncol 2012;109(2):301–7.

64. Sant M, Minicozzi P, Lagorio S, et al. Survival of European patients with central nervous system tumors. Int J Cancer 2012;131(1):173–85.

65. Tseng MY, Tseng JH, Merchant E. Comparison of effects of socioeconomic and geographic variations on survival for adults and children with glioma. J Neurosurg 2006;105(4 Suppl):297–305.

66. Crocetti E, Trama A, Stiller C, et al. Epidemiology of glial and non-glial brain tumours in Europe. Eur J Cancer 2012;48(10):1532–42.

67. Claus EB, Black PM. Survival rates and patterns of care for patients diagnosed with supratentorial low-grade gliomas: data from the SEER program, 1973-2001. Cancer 2006;106(6):1358–63.

68. Pignatti F, van den Bent M, Curran D, et al. Prognostic factors for survival in adult patients with cerebral low-grade glioma. J Clin Oncol 2002;20(8):2076–84.

69. Pallud J, Audureau E, Blonski M, et al. Epileptic seizures in diffuse low-grade gliomas in adults. Brain 2014;137(Pt 2):449–62.

70. Chang EF, Clark A, Jensen RL, et al. Multiinstitutional validation of the University of California at San Francisco low-grade glioma prognostic scoring system. Clinical article. J Neurosurg 2009;111(2):203–10.

71. Capelle L, Fontaine D, Mandonnet E, et al. Spontaneous and therapeutic prognostic factors in adult hemispheric World Health Organization Grade II gliomas: a series of 1097 cases: clinical article. J Neurosurg 2013;118(6):1157–68.

72. Pallud J, Blonski M, Mandonnet E, et al. Velocity of tumor spontaneous expansion predicts long-term outcomes for diffuse low-grade gliomas. Neuro Oncol 2013;15(5):595–606.

73. Yan H, Parsons DW, Jin G, et al. IDH1 and IDH2 mutations in gliomas. N Engl J Med 2009;360(8):765–73.

74. Hartmann C, Hentschel B, Tatagiba M, et al. Molecular markers in low-grade gliomas: predictive or prognostic? Clin Cancer Res 2011;17(13):4588–99.

75. Smith JS, Perry A, Borell TJ, et al. Alterations of chromosome arms 1p and 19q as predictors of survival in oligodendrogliomas, astrocytomas, and mixed oligoastrocytomas. J Clin Oncol 2000;18(3):636–45.

76. Okamoto Y, Di Patre PL, Burkhard C, et al. Population-based study on incidence, survival rates, and genetic alterations of low-grade diffuse

astrocytomas and oligodendrogliomas. Acta Neuropathol 2004;108(1):49–56.

77. Jakola AS, Myrmel KS, Kloster R, et al. Comparison of a strategy favoring early surgical resection vs a strategy favoring watchful waiting in low-grade gliomas. JAMA 2012;308(18):1881–8.

78. Sanai N, Chang S, Berger MS. Low-grade gliomas in adults. J Neurosurg 2011;115(5):948–65.

79. Duffau H. A new philosophy in surgery for diffuse low-grade glioma (DLGG): oncological and functional outcomes. Neurochirurgie 2013;59(1):2–8.

80. Ramakrishna R, Hebb A, Barber J, et al. Outcomes in reoperated low-grade gliomas. Neurosurgery 2015;77(2):175–84 [discussion: 184].

81. Buckner JC, Shaw EG, Pugh SL, et al. Radiation plus procarbazine, CCNU, and vincristine in low-grade glioma. N Engl J Med 2016;374(14): 1344–55.

82. Weller M, van den Bent M, Tonn JC, et al. European Association for Neuro-Oncology (EANO) guideline on the diagnosis and treatment of adult astrocytic and oligodendroglial gliomas. Lancet Oncol 2017; 18(6):e315–29.

83. Jhaveri J, Liu Y, Chowdhary M, et al. Is less more? Comparing chemotherapy alone with chemotherapy and radiation for high-risk grade 2 glioma: an analysis of the National Cancer Data Base. Cancer 2018;124(6):1169–78.

84. Bady P, Kurscheid S, Delorenzi M, et al. The DNA methylome of DDR genes and benefit from RT or TMZ in IDH mutant low-grade glioma treated in EORTC 22033. Acta Neuropathol 2018;135(4): 601–15.

85. Mandonnet E, Duffau H. An attempt to conceptualize the individual onco-functional balance: Why a standardized treatment is an illusion for diffuse low-grade glioma patients. Crit Rev Oncol Hematol 2018;122:83–91.

86. Duffau H, Taillandier L. New concepts in the management of diffuse low-grade glioma: proposal of a multistage and individualized therapeutic approach. Neuro Oncol 2015;17(3):332–42.

87. Sanson M, Hosking FJ, Shete S, et al. Chromosome 7p11.2 (EGFR) variation influences glioma risk. Hum Mol Genet 2011;20(14):2897–904.

88. Enciso-Mora V, Hosking FJ, Kinnersley B, et al. Deciphering the 8q24.21 association for glioma. Hum Mol Genet 2013;22(11):2293–302.

89. Rice T, Zheng S, Decker PA, et al. Inherited variant on chromosome 11q23 increases susceptibility to IDH-mutated but not IDH-normal gliomas regardless of grade or histology. Neuro Oncol 2013;15(5): 535–41.

90. Stacey SN, Sulem P, Jonasdottir A, et al. A germline variant in the TP53 polyadenylation signal confers cancer susceptibility. Nat Genet 2011;43(11):1098–103.

91. Enciso-Mora V, Hosking FJ, Di Stefano AL, et al. Low penetrance susceptibility to glioma is caused by the TP53 variant rs78378222. Br J Cancer 2013;108(10): 2178–85.

Molecular Pathogenesis of Low-Grade Glioma

Devin Bready, BS[a], Dimitris G. Placantonakis, MD, PhD[b],*

KEYWORDS

- Low-grade glioma • Astrocytoma • Oligodendroglioma • Mutant IDH

KEY POINTS

- Recent advances in genome sequencing have identified genetic alterations that define low-grade glioma.
- The isocitrate dehydrogenase mutation initiates metabolic, epigenetic, and cellular changes that transform neural progenitors to glioma cells.
- Laboratory findings are giving rise to novel therapeutic approaches in low-grade glioma.

INTRODUCTION

Gliomas represent the most common primary brain tumor in adults. Low-grade gliomas (LGGs) are indolent tumors that almost universally progress to high-grade secondary aggressive tumors, such as glioblastoma. The time course of progression can vary greatly from as little as 2 years to greater than a decade depending on the molecular features and the location of the LGG within the brain. The clinical course of LGG is generally less aggressive than primary glioblastoma and its incidence peaks at an earlier age, during the third and fourth decades of life, as opposed to most glioblastoma cases, which peak in the sixth to seventh decades.[1–3] Understanding of the relatedness and uniqueness of these 2 entities has undergone a revolution during the past decade with the advent of widespread cancer genome sequencing. Although clinicians at one time relied only on pathologic grade and morphologic features to classify tumors and inform treatment, genomic sequencing of gliomas has generated a paradigm shift in the approach to understanding and treating the disease. In 2009, it was discovered that the vast majority of LGG harbored mutations in isocitrate dehydrogenase (IDH) 1 and less frequently in the closely related enzyme IDH2.[4]

The research community is still in the relatively early stages of transforming the basic scientific advances of the last decade into novel therapeutics. This article discusses molecular and cellular mechanisms underlying LGG pathogenesis and progression to high-grade tumors as well as potential therapeutic approaches that have emerged from laboratory findings.

MOLECULAR ALTERATIONS IN ADULT LOW-GRADE GLIOMAS

In 2009, LGG and secondary glioblastoma, which originates from a preexisting LGG, were shown to harbor characteristic, neomorphic, heterozygous mutations in IDH1.[4] This cytosolic, NADP$^+$-dependent enzyme normally forms a homodimer and takes part in the conversion of isocitrate to α-ketoglutarate (α-KG), which can then be used for multiple cellular functions.[5] Additionally, LGGs lacking a mutation in IDH1 may harbor an analogous mutation in IDH2, a mitochondrial enzyme

Disclosure Statement: Dr. Bready was supported by (NIH T32GM007308 and Dr. Placantonakis got support from NY State Stem Cell Program - DOH01-STEM5-2016-00221 and NIH/NINDS R01 NS102665.

[a] Department of Neurosurgery, NYU School of Medicine, 530 First Avenue, Skirball 8R, New York, NY 10016, USA; [b] Department of Neurosurgery, Kimmel Center for Stem Cell Biology, Laura and Isaac Perlmutter Cancer Center, Neuroscience Institute, Brain Tumor Center, NYU School of Medicine, 530 First Avenue, Skirball 8R, New York, NY 10016, USA
* Corresponding author.
E-mail address: dimitris.placantonakis@nyumc.org

Neurosurg Clin N Am 30 (2019) 17–25
https://doi.org/10.1016/j.nec.2018.08.011
1042-3680/19/© 2018 The Author(s). Published by Elsevier Inc. This is an open access article under the CC BY-NC-ND license (http://creativecommons.org/licenses/by-nc-nd/4.0/).

that also produces α-KG, primarily for the tricarboxylic acid (TCA) cycle.[1] LGG and secondary glioblastomas are not the only contexts in which these mutations are found. Acute myeloid leukemia, cholangiocarcinoma, and myelodysplastic syndromes have been found to exhibit the same class of mutations.[6,7] The genetic syndrome Ollier disease, which results from somatic mosaicism for mutations in IDH, is associated with an increased rate of gliomas compared with the general population and an earlier age of diagnosis than seen in the broader LGG patient population.[8,9]

After their initial identification in LGG and secondary glioblastoma, IDH mutations were identified in greater than 80% of tumors histologically classified as LGG.[4,10] Further analysis of genomic sequencing revealed the presence of 2 distinct molecular subclasses within LGG (**Fig. 1**). The larger of these subclasses is characterized by inactivating mutations in the tumor suppressor TP53 and the chromatin remodeling enzyme ATRX (see **Fig. 1**).[2,10] Tumors containing this set of mutations correspond to astrocytoma, as identified by histopathology.[11] The smaller subclass is characterized by codeletion of chromosome 1p/19q and promoter mutations in telomerase reverse transcriptase (*TERT*) (see **Fig. 1**B).[11] This latter group of tumors corresponds to oligodendroglioma. IDH mutant and P53/ATRX mutated (astrocytic) LGG has a more aggressive clinical course.[11] Although IDH mutant 1p/19q codeleted glioma (oligodendroglioma) shows a less aggressive behavior, significant neurologic deterioration and mortality do occur.[12,13]

All of this classification so far neglects the small percentage of histopathologically graded LGGs, which do not exhibit a mutation in IDH1/2. It has been suggested that these IDH wild-type gliomas essentially behave like glioblastoma. If looking for markers of IDH wild-type glioblastoma (epidermal growth factor receptor amplification, H3F3A K27M, or *TERT* promoter mutation), they can be found in approximately half of these patients.[14] These patients have an average survival of 1.23 years, comparable to glioblastoma. The other half of IDH wild-type LGGs, however, lack these mutations and have a clinical course resembling more closely that of LGG, with average survival of greater than 7 years.[13,14]

The most recent update to the World Health Organization guidelines on the classification of central nervous system tumors released in 2016 has incorporated the molecular features, discussed previously, into the classification of adult LGG. Histopathology remains vital in first diagnosing a tumor as a diffuse glioma and then in determining tumor grade. If a tumor is determined to be a diffuse glioma and grade II or III, then molecular diagnostics dictate further classifications. The presence of a mutation in IDH1/2 in combination with loss of ATRX and TP53 results in the diagnosis of a diffuse astrocytoma or anaplastic astrocytoma, grade II and grade III, respectively.[11] If IDH mutations are found in combination with chromosomal 1p/19q codeletion, then a diagnosis of oligodendroglioma or anaplastic oligodendroglioma is made.[11] A diagnosis of oligoastrocytoma, previously defined as a tumor with both astrocytic and oligodendroglial histology, still exists in the updated guidelines but is much less common by the new definition. Oligoastrocytomas now must possess distinct tumor cell populations with the molecular features of both astrocytoma and oligodendroglioma, but these are exceedingly rare.[15] Finally, those tumors that are histologically grade II or grade III and lack mutations in the previously discussed genes are grouped by histology into either IDH wild-type astrocytoma or oligodendroglioma not otherwise specified.[11]

MOLECULAR PATHOGENESIS OF LOW-GRADE ASTROCYTOMA

Patient genomic analysis established the mutations, discussed previously, as being nearly pathognomonic for low-grade astrocytoma (LGA) and low-grade oliodendroglioma (LGO), but studying how each individual mutation or combination of mutations contribute to tumorigenesis is important for making this information therapeutically actionable. It was previously recognized that a fraction of glioblastomas and a majority of LGG shared a genome-wide pattern of increased DNA methylation, termed *glioma-CpG island methylator phenotype* (*G-CIMP*).[16] The best studied consequence of DNA methylation is the silencing of gene expression when gene promoter regions are methylated.[17] The effects, however, do not stop here. High levels of methylation have been linked to heightened mutagenesis in colorectal cancer, another malignancy where many tumors exhibit increased CpG island methylation.[18] Beyond modifying gene promoter activity, genomic methylation can affect expression by altering chromatin organization.[19–22] Although the exact consequences of the G-CIMP phenotype are not clear, analysis of the actions of mutant IDH provided a mechanistic link to its establishment.

Evidence for IDH mutations as a driver of gliomagenesis was supported by their presence in several distinct glioma subtypes and other tumors, but the strongest evidence was seen in studies of IDH-mutant glioma recurrences after initial treatment.[23] It has been convincingly shown that if an initial tumor contains a mutant IDH, then 100% of

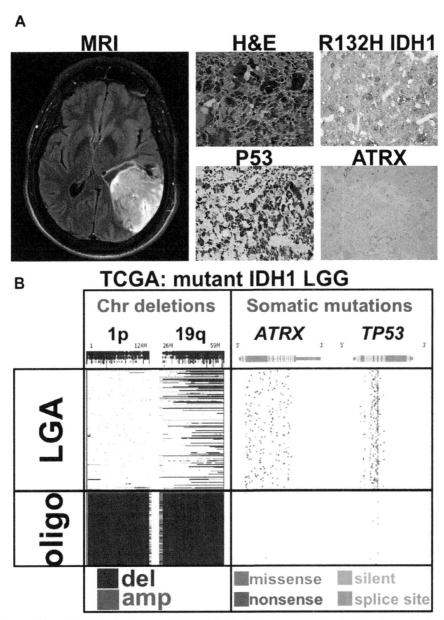

Fig. 1. Radiographic and histologic features of LGG. (*A*) The MRI shows a patient with a large, brain-infiltrating IDH mutant astrocytoma. At the histologic level, tumor cells were positive for the R132H IDH1 mutation; P53 nuclear staining, suggesting loss-of-function mutation; and loss of ATRX. H&E, hematoxylin and eosin staining × original magnification × 20. (*B*) Analysis of genetic profile of IDH1 mutant LGGs in the TCGA. LGAs and oligodendrogliomas (oligo) have mutually exclusive genetic changes. LGAs are characterized by loss-of-function TP53 and ATRX mutations, and do not show the 1p/19q codeletion seen in oligodendrogliomas.

recurrences also contain the same exact mutation.[23] This strongly supports the hypothesis that mutations in IDH1/2 are the driving event behind the formation of an IDH mutant LGG and remain necessary for tumor progression.

As discussed previously, IDH1 is a cytosolic enzyme that catalyzes the conversion of isocitrate to α-KG, which is then used for multiple metabolic purposes and is required by a class of enzymes

called dioxygenases for catalytic activity (**Fig. 2A**).[24] Among these enzymes, some are responsible for removing chromatin methylation, on both DNA and histones.[25,26] IDH2 is a homologous enzyme found in the mitochondria and produces α-KG for use in the TCA cycle, a process necessary for aerobic metabolism and ATP production. In contrast, the neomorphic IDH mutations produce the unique metabolic product 2-

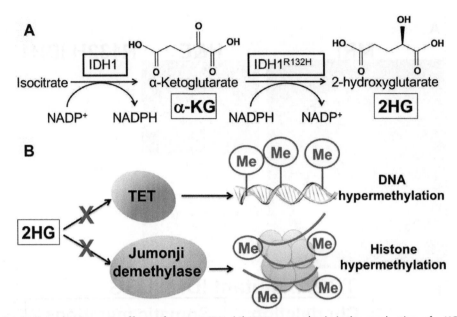

Fig. 2. Metabolic and epigenetic effects of mutant IDH. (*A*) IDH's normal role is the production of α-KG, a metabolic intermediate necessary for catalytic activity of enzymes that include ten-eleven translocases (TET), which initiate DNA demethylation, and Jumonji histone demethylases. (*B*) The oncogenic production of 2HG directly inhibits such enzymes, leading to DNA and histone hypermethylation. Me, Methyl Group.

hydroxyglutarate (2HG),[27] which inhibits dioxygenase catalytic activity, resulting in DNA hypermethylation among other effects (see **Fig. 2**).[25] Studies have confirmed that mutant IDH is sufficient to impart the G-CIMP DNA hypermethylation epigenotype seen in patients.[25] Furthermore, mutant IDH increases histone methylation, in particular repressive methylation modifications associated with transcriptionally silent chromatin.[28]

LGAs, as discussed previously, harbor inactivating mutations of *TP53* and *ATRX*. P53 is a stereotypical tumor suppressor whose inactivation is observed in 50% of all human cancers.[29] Its ability to halt cell-cycle progression in response to cellular stresses, including DNA damage, makes it a central player in the preservation of genome integrity and prevention of tumorigenic alterations. Without its activity cells can accumulate extensive mutations and genomic damage while still progressing through the cell cycle, producing progeny containing those errors. Individuals lacking 1 of the 2 alleles for *TP53* in Li-Fraumeni syndrome are at remarkably increased risk for developing several tumors through loss of heterozygosity.[30]

The function of ATRX is not as clear as P53. ATRX is mutated less often than P53 in cancers, but similar inactivating mutations have been identified in LGG, neuroendocrine tumors of the pancreas, neuroblastoma, and osteosarcoma among others.[31] ATRX is one of many chromatin remodeling enzymes belonging to the SWI/SNF family.[32] Chromatin, the complex of DNA and

proteins in the nucleus, is reversibly modified in several ways to alter how accessible areas of the genome are for the purposes of regulating gene expression.[32] In particular, ARTX modulates chromatin found near a cell's telomeres, repeating regions of DNA at the ends of chromosomes.[32,33] When ATRX is inactivated, as in LGA, cells begin to undergo a process, termed *alternative lengthening of telomeres (ALT)*.[34,35] Telomeres shorten with each round of cellular division and thus the replicative life span of cells is limited by the length of their telomeres. The prototypical method of circumventing this limitation is the expression of telomerase, as in embryonic stem cells, which preserves telomere length, whereas in certain types of cancer lacking ATRX the ALT mechanism is deployed.[36] Inactivation of ATRX has also been observed to contribute to the invasive, migratory phenotype of glioma cells both by itself and in the presence of mutant IDH and loss of P53.[22,37] The loss of ATRX in laboratory models is associated with drastic changes in gene expression profiles mirroring those seen human LGA specimens.[37]

Despite these insights into mutant IDH1 gliomagenesis, the exact mechanism whereby the mutation transforms neural cells into glioma remains unclear.[38,39] Limited understanding of the disease process is in large part related to lack of patient-derived xenograft models that recapitulate the disease, due to the inability of LGGs to grow in culture ex vivo. To overcome this limitation and elucidate cellular and molecular mechanisms of

LGG pathogenesis, the authors recently developed a novel LGG model that is based on a human neural stem cell (hNSC) platform.[22] The authors derived these hNSCs from human embryonic stem cells and genetically engineered them to express mutant IDH1 (the R132H mutation) as well as short hairpin RNAs that specifically knockdown P53 and ATRX, to mimic the stereotypic genetic background of LGA. Although these 3 genetic alterations did not alter cellular proliferation rates, they blocked the ability of hNSCs to differentiate into postmitotic neuronal and glial lineages (**Fig. 3A**), similar to what others have described[26,28,40]; enabled ALT-dependent telomere elongation (**Fig. 3B**); and enhanced their ability to infiltrate normal brain tissue (**Fig. 3C**), a hallmark of LGA. The authors' findings suggest that the oncogenic mechanism underlying LGG genesis is the prevention of generation of postmitotic neuroglial lineages from brain progenitor cells by the combination of mutant IDH and loss of P53 and ATRX, resulting in the slow growth of undifferentiated, proliferating stemlike tumor cells.[22]

What was even more fascinating, however, was the molecular mechanism the authors demonstrated that underlies this differentiation block. SOX2 is a transcription factor that is crucial in maintaining the ability of hNSCs to differentiate to neuroglial lineages. The authors found that SOX2 became transcriptionally down-regulated in hNSCs bearing mutant IDH1 and loss of P53/ATRX (**Fig. 4A**) amid other massive transcriptome changes initiated by the 3 hits. The authors showed the change in SOX2 expression is necessary and sufficient for the differentiation block, a finding suggesting SOX2 acts as an atypical tumor suppressor during LGA initiation. The authors also confirmed the change in SOX2 expression between normal human brain tissue and IDH mutant LGA (**Fig. 4B**). This transcriptional silencing of SOX2 was not due to hypermethylation of its promoter. Instead, the authors' evidence suggests that this effect is mediated by unfolding of the normal chromatin conformation, leading to disassociation of the SOX2 promoter from putative distal enhancer elements located 600 kb to 700 kb downstream of the SOX2 locus. The authors believe the chromatin conformational changes are due to reduced occupancy of CTCF, a protein that helps organize chromatin folding, at its motifs within this genomic neighborhood, partly due to increased DNA methylation (**Fig. 4C**). This mechanism is similar to one reported in high-grade IDH mutated gliomas.[21] More specifically, Flavahan and colleagues[21] found reduced CTCF occupancy leading to abnormal chromatin folding and demonstrated that, as a consequence, a proto-

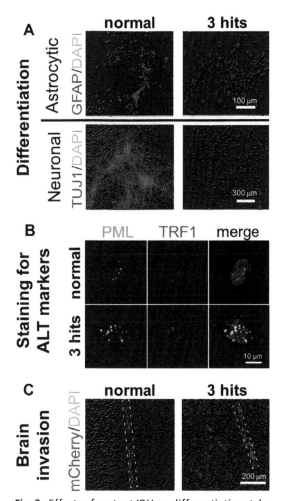

Fig. 3. Effects of mutant IDH on differentiation, telomere elongation, and brain invasion. (*A*) Although normal hNSCs can be directed to differentiate to neurons and astrocytes (*left*) as shown by strong Neuron-specific Class III β-tubulin (TUJ1) staining or Glial Fibrillary Acidic Protein (GFAP) staining respectively, hNSCs with 3 genetic alterations found in LGA (3 hits) show a differentiation block as evidenced by the lack of TUJ1 staining or GFAP staining (*right*). (*B*) At 63× magnification the nuclei of hNSCs with 3 hits demonstrate foci in which staining for PML and TRF1 colocalize (*yellow*), indicating ALT, whereas normal hNSCs do not. (*C*) Injection of normal or 3-hit hNSCs expressing the fluorescent protein mCherry into the brain of immunosuppressed (NOD.SCID) mice reveals a significant increase in brain invasion by 3-hit cells. The dotted lines outline the injection tracks. In all images, nuclei were counterstained with DAPI. (*Adapted from* Modrek AS, Golub D, Khan T, et al. Low-grade astrocytoma mutations in IDH1, P53, and ATRX cooperate to block differentiation of human neural stem cells via repression of SOX2. Cell Rep 2017;21(5):1271; with permission.)

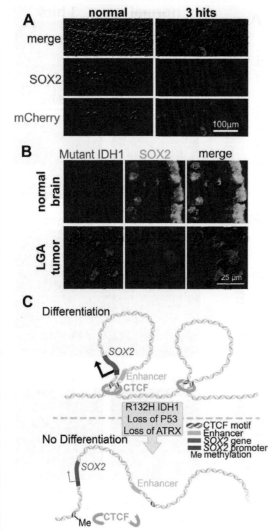

Fig. 4. Mutant IDH alters chromatin conformation in LGA initiation. (*A*) Confocal microscopic images of hNSCs expressing mCherry injected in the mouse brain. The expression of transcription factor SOX2 is down-regulated in 3-hit versus normal hNSCs. (*B*) Similar to the authors' hNSC model, actual mutant IDH1 LGA tumors show reduced SOX2 × original magnification × 40 expression relative to native neural progenitor cells in the subventricular zone of the normal adult brain. (*C*) Schematic illustrating how methylation of CTCF motifs due to mutant IDH alters chromatin conformation, leading to disassociation of *SOX2* promoter from an enhancer and reduced *SOX2* transcription. In all images, nuclei were counterstained with DAPI. (*Adapted from* Modrek AS, Golub D, Khan T, et al. Low-grade astrocytoma mutations in IDH1, P53, and ATRX cooperate to block differentiation of human neural stem cells via repression of SOX2. Cell Rep 2017;21(5):1267–80; with permission.)

oncogene, *PDGFRA*, became overexpressed due to ectopic transcriptional activation by an enhancer that it normally does not interact with. These findings illustrate the important contribution of altered chromatin conformation to the pathogenesis of LGA.

MOLECULAR PATHOGENESIS OF LOW-GRADE OLIGODENDROGLIOMA

LGOs make up a relatively smaller portion of LGGs and are not as well studied as astrocytomas. Mutations in IDH are near universal in LGO and the consequences of this change is much the same as it is in LGA. The pathognomonic molecular changes in LGO are the chromosomal deletion of 1p and 19q and mutations in the promoter of *TERT*.[2] Hemizygous codeletion of chromosome arms 1p and 19q results in the loss of several genes. *TERT* promoter mutations, resulting in overexpression of TERT, provide a mechanism by which tumors can maintain telomere length and avoid replicative senescence.[41]

Beyond the 2 hallmark changes discussed previously, LGO harbors inactivating mutations of the homolog of capicua (*CIC*) and far-upstream binding protein 1 (*FUBP1*) in 70% and 30% of cases, respectively.[42] These 2 genes are found on chromosomal segments 1p (*FUBP1*) and 19q (*CIC*), so that additional inactivating mutations in the context of 1p/19q codeletion result in complete loss of these proteins. Loss of CIC, a transcriptional repressor, was recently found to promote the proliferation and block the differentiation of neural progenitors,[43] thus providing a mechanism for oligodendroglioma initiation and growth. FUBP1 mutations are less well characterized but seem to result in transcriptional activation of C-MYC, a transcription factor activated by growth factor signaling, and up-regulation of ribosome biogenesis.[12,44] Additionally, in normal physiology FUBP1 promotes neural differentiation of progenitor cells.[45]

PROGRESSION TO HIGH-GRADE GLIOMA

Mutant IDH LGA and LGO both inevitably progress to high-grade gliomas. A recent study was able to catalog genetic changes underlying this progression by performing whole-exome sequencing on LGGs resected on initial presentation and after their transformation to high-grade tumors.[23] The most common deletion associated with progression was that of tumor suppressor *CDKN2A*, whereas the most common amplification was that of *MYC*.[23] Additionally, the majority of tumors overexpressed *EZH2* on progression.[23] EZH2 is the catalytic subunit of the polycomb repressive complex 2 (PRC2) and catalyzes the trimethylation of lysine 27 on histone H3.[46] This histone modification is associated with transcriptional repression.[47] This finding again suggests a crucial role for regulation of the epigenome in the pathogenesis of IDH mutant glioma.

It has been demonstrated that treatment of IDH mutant LGG with the alkylating agent temozolomide generates a hypermutant genotype in 60% of cases.[48] This increased mutational burden is associated with exacerbated malignancy. In contrast, only approximately 20% of IDH wild-type gliomas respond to chemotherapy with this hypermutation phenomenon.[49] Common genetic alterations in the acquisition of the hypermutant genotype include loss of CDKN2A and mutations to other components of the RB tumor suppressor pathway as well as several of the components of the MAPK signaling pathway.[48]

THERAPEUTIC IMPLICATIONS

As with other tumors of the central nervous system, treatment of LGG continues to rely on maximal tumor resection, radiation, and cytotoxic chemotherapy. Modern understanding of the unique pathogenic causes of LGG, however, has spawned several experimental approaches to treatment that show promise.

Inhibition of Mutant Isocitrate Dehydrogenase 1/2

Several inhibitors of mutant IDH have been produced and their use in treating several cancers is now under investigation. These drugs have been validated to specifically inhibit 2HG but not α-KG production. Early clinical data in IDH mutant acute myeloid leukemia have shown promise. The Food and Drug Administration approved the first compound in late 2017 for this indication.[50] Trials in glioma are ongoing due to the longer timeline of the disease. Early preclinical evidence showed promise that inhibitors could slow tumor progression.[51] Later studies have indicated, however, that inhibitors have no inhibitory effect on tumor growth in xenoplant models of glioma despite effective inhibition of 2HG production.[52] Current evidence shows that the effects of mutant IDH are long-lasting and remain even after full inhibition of 2HG production. Several genes, whose expression is changed by 2HG, remain aberrantly expressed after prolonged inhibition of mutant IDH.[53]

Synthetic Lethality in Low-Grade Glioma

A growing area of interest in oncology is finding ways in which oncogenic mutations cause cells to become overly reliant on pathways that healthy cells use but can survive without. If such a pathway is found, targeted interference in its function can eliminate cancerous cells while sparing their healthy counterparts. Using tractable laboratory models of LGG, several such vulnerabilities have been identified.

One of the most potentially disastrous types of DNA damage that cells can incur are DNA breaks. When these breaks occur in healthy cells in the S and G2 phases of the cell cycle, the preferred mechanism of repair is to use the homologous sister chromatid as a template.[54] This high-fidelity mechanism of DNA repair is termed, *homologous recombination repair* (*HRR*), and preserves genomic integrity. A different and somewhat less effective mechanism, nonhomologous end joining (NHEJ), is theoretically available for repair throughout the cell cycle but acts primarily in G1 as a result of its suppression in S/G2 by proteins like CYREN.[55] Finally, the most error-prone DNA repair mechanism, alternative end-joining (Alt-EJ), is dependent on poly (ADP-ribose) polymerase (PARP) and serves as backup when HRR and NHEJ are not available.[56] Lack of repair of DNA breaks by any mechanism results in cell death.

In 2016, Sulkowski and colleagues[57] showed that IDH mutant LGG harbors a defect in HRR and is inherently susceptible to PARP inhibitors because it relies on Alt-EJ for DNA repair. This mechanism was previously identified and understood in BRCA1/2-deficient breast cancer and led to the development of PARP inhibitors.[58] Clinical trials have already begun to assess the efficacy of PARP inhibitors in mutant IDH glioma.

Another effect of mutant IDH is to reduce cellular nicotinamide adenine dinucleotide (NAD$^+$) levels by transcriptionally down-regulating the NAD$^+$ salvage pathway enzyme nicotinate phosphoribosyltransferase (NARPT1).[52] Preclinical animal model testing has found strong sensitivity of mutant IDH glioma to NAD$^+$ depletion via inhibition of nicotinamide phosphoribosyltransferase (NAMPT), the sole enzyme that can support NAD$^+$ biosynthesis in the absence of NARPT1.[52] This finding uncovered a metabolic vulnerability of IDH mutant glioma that can be therapeutically exploited.

Cells express proteins that inhibit or activate apoptosis in a context-dependent manner. It was recently demonstrated that mutant IDH can change the balance of these factors.[59] The presence of mutant IDH or exogenous 2HG activates the energy-sensing protein AMP-activated protein kinase, which has the downstream effect of inhibiting production of MCL1,[59] a member of the Bcl-2/Bcl-xL antiapoptotic family of proteins.[60] Because of the low levels of MCL1, treatment of mutant IDH glioma with the compound ABT263, which is an inhibitor of Bcl-xL and Bcl-2, depletes

IDH mutant tumor cells of antiapoptotic activity and confers synthetic lethality with the IDH mutation both in vitro and in vivo.[59] This fascinating finding also exposed another selective vulnerability of IDH mutant gliomas not seen in their wild-type counterparts.

SUMMARY

In the past decade, much has been learned about LGG molecular pathogenesis. Currently, there are significant efforts to translate this knowledge into clinical trials. The IDH mutation, a hallmark of LGG, is important to understand further to be therapeutically targeted. Recent studies are revealing unique vulnerabilities in IDH mutant glioma, which may soon bring forth clinically impactful treatments.

REFERENCES

1. Grier JT, Batchelor T. Low-grade gliomas in adults. Oncologist 2006;11(6):681–93.
2. Cancer Genome Atlas Research N, Brat DJ, Verhaak RG, et al. Comprehensive, integrative genomic analysis of diffuse lower-grade gliomas. N Engl J Med 2015;372(26):2481–98.
3. Ceccarelli M, Barthel FP, Malta TM, et al. Molecular profiling reveals biologically discrete subsets and pathways of progression in diffuse glioma. Cell 2016;164(3):550–63.
4. Yan H, Parsons DW, Jin G, et al. IDH1 and IDH2 mutations in gliomas. N Engl J Med 2009;360(8):765–73.
5. Vinekar R, Verma C, Ghosh I. Functional relevance of dynamic properties of Dimeric NADP-dependent Isocitrate Dehydrogenases. BMC Bioinformatics 2012;13(Suppl 17):S2.
6. Farshidfar F, Zheng S, Gingras MC, et al. Integrative genomic analysis of cholangiocarcinoma identifies distinct IDH-mutant molecular profiles. Cell Rep 2017;19(13):2878–80.
7. Yen KE, Bittinger MA, Su SM, et al. Cancer-associated IDH mutations: biomarker and therapeutic opportunities. Oncogene 2010;29(49):6409–17.
8. Bonnet C, Thomas L, Psimaras D, et al. Characteristics of gliomas in patients with somatic IDH mosaicism. Acta Neuropathol Commun 2016;4:31.
9. Amary MF, Damato S, Halai D, et al. Ollier disease and Maffucci syndrome are caused by somatic mosaic mutations of IDH1 and IDH2. Nat Genet 2011;43(12):1262–5.
10. Balss J, Meyer J, Mueller W, et al. Analysis of the IDH1 codon 132 mutation in brain tumors. Acta Neuropathol 2008;116(6):597–602.
11. Louis DN, Perry A, Reifenberger G, et al. The 2016 World Health Organization classification of tumors of the central nervous system: a summary. Acta Neuropathol 2016;131(6):803–20.
12. Wesseling P, van den Bent M, Perry A. Oligodendroglioma: pathology, molecular mechanisms and markers. Acta Neuropathol 2015;129(6):809–27.
13. Bromberg JE, van den Bent MJ. Oligodendrogliomas: molecular biology and treatment. Oncologist 2009;14(2):155–63.
14. Aibaidula A, Chan AK, Shi Z, et al. Adult IDH wild-type lower-grade gliomas should be further stratified. Neuro Oncol 2017;19(10):1327–37.
15. Huse JT, Diamond EL, Wang L, et al. Mixed glioma with molecular features of composite oligodendroglioma and astrocytoma: a true "oligoastrocytoma"? Acta Neuropathol 2015;129(1):151–3.
16. Noushmehr H, Weisenberger DJ, Diefes K, et al. Identification of a CpG island methylator phenotype that defines a distinct subgroup of glioma. Cancer Cell 2010;17(5):510–22.
17. McGhee JD, Ginder GD. Specific DNA methylation sites in the vicinity of the chicken beta-globin genes. Nature 1979;280(5721):419–20.
18. Weisenberger DJ, Siegmund KD, Campan M, et al. CpG island methylator phenotype underlies sporadic microsatellite instability and is tightly associated with BRAF mutation in colorectal cancer. Nat Genet 2006;38(7):787–93.
19. Gilbert N, Thomson I, Boyle S, et al. DNA methylation affects nuclear organization, histone modifications, and linker histone binding but not chromatin compaction. J Cell Biol 2007;177(3):401–11.
20. Keshet I, Lieman-Hurwitz J, Cedar H. DNA methylation affects the formation of active chromatin. Cell 1986;44(4):535–43.
21. Flavahan WA, Drier Y, Liau BB, et al. Insulator dysfunction and oncogene activation in IDH mutant gliomas. Nature 2016;529(7584):110–4.
22. Modrek AS, Golub D, Khan T, et al. Low-grade astrocytoma mutations in IDH1, P53, and ATRX cooperate to block differentiation of human neural stem cells via repression of SOX2. Cell Rep 2017;21(5):1267–80.
23. Bai H, Harmanci AS, Erson-Omay EZ, et al. Integrated genomic characterization of IDH1-mutant glioma malignant progression. Nat Genet 2016;48(1):59–66.
24. Xu W, Yang H, Liu Y, et al. Oncometabolite 2-hydroxyglutarate is a competitive inhibitor of alpha-ketoglutarate-dependent dioxygenases. Cancer Cell 2011;19(1):17–30.
25. Turcan S, Rohle D, Goenka A, et al. IDH1 mutation is sufficient to establish the glioma hypermethylator phenotype. Nature 2012;483(7390):479–83.
26. Figueroa ME, Abdel-Wahab O, Lu C, et al. Leukemic IDH1 and IDH2 mutations result in a hypermethylation phenotype, disrupt TET2 function, and impair hematopoietic differentiation. Cancer Cell 2010; 18(6):553–67.
27. Dang L, White DW, Gross S, et al. Cancer-associated IDH1 mutations produce 2-hydroxyglutarate. Nature 2009;462(7274):739–44.

28. Lu C, Ward PS, Kapoor GS, et al. IDH mutation impairs histone demethylation and results in a block to cell differentiation. Nature 2012;483(7390):474–8.

29. Vogelstein B, Lane D, Levine AJ. Surfing the p53 network. Nature 2000;408(6810):307–10.

30. McBride KA, Ballinger ML, Killick E, et al. Li-Fraumeni syndrome: cancer risk assessment and clinical management. Nat Rev Clin Oncol 2014;11(5):260–71.

31. Fishbein L, Khare S, Wubbenhorst B, et al. Whole-exome sequencing identifies somatic ATRX mutations in pheochromocytomas and paragangliomas. Nat Commun 2015;6:6140.

32. Clynes D, Higgs DR, Gibbons RJ. The chromatin remodeller ATRX: a repeat offender in human disease. Trends Biochem Sci 2013;38(9):461–6.

33. Wong LH, McGhie JD, Sim M, et al. ATRX interacts with H3.3 in maintaining telomere structural integrity in pluripotent embryonic stem cells. Genome Res 2010;20(3):351–60.

34. Napier CE, Huschtscha LI, Harvey A, et al. ATRX represses alternative lengthening of telomeres. Oncotarget 2015;6(18):16543–58.

35. Mukherjee J, Johannessen TA, Ohba S, et al. Mutant IDH1 cooperates with ATRX loss to drive the alternative lengthening of telomere (ALT) phenotype in glioma. Cancer Res 2018;78(11):2966–77.

36. Dilley RL, Greenberg RA. ALTernative telomere maintenance and cancer. Trends Cancer 2015;1(2):145–56.

37. Danussi C, Bose P, Parthasarathy PT, et al. Atrx inactivation drives disease-defining phenotypes in glioma cells of origin through global epigenomic remodeling. Nat Commun 2018;9(1):1057.

38. Bardella C, Al-Dalahmah O, Krell D, et al. Expression of Idh1(R132H) in the Murine subventricular zone stem cell niche recapitulates features of early gliomagenesis. Cancer Cell 2016;30(4):578–94.

39. Pirozzi CJ, Carpenter AB, Waitkus MS, et al. Mutant IDH1 disrupts the mouse subventricular zone and alters brain tumor progression. Mol Cancer Res 2017;15(5):507–20.

40. Rosiak K, Smolarz M, Stec WJ, et al. IDH1R132H in neural stem cells: differentiation impaired by increased apoptosis. PLoS One 2016;11(5):e0154726.

41. Walsh KM, Wiencke JK, Lachance DH, et al. Telomere maintenance and the etiology of adult glioma. Neuro Oncol 2015;17(11):1445–52.

42. Bettegowda C, Agrawal N, Jiao Y, et al. Mutations in CIC and FUBP1 contribute to human oligodendroglioma. Science 2011;333(6048):1453–5.

43. Yang R, Chen LH, Hansen LJ, et al. Cic loss promotes gliomagenesis via aberrant neural stem cell proliferation and differentiation. Cancer Res 2017;77(22):6097–108.

44. He L, Liu J, Collins I, et al. Loss of FBP function arrests cellular proliferation and extinguishes c-myc expression. EMBO J 2000;19(5):1034–44.

45. Hwang I, Cao D, Na Y, et al. Far upstream element-binding protein 1 regulates LSD1 alternative splicing to promote terminal differentiation of neural progenitors. Stem Cell Reports 2018;10(4):1208–21.

46. Margueron R, Reinberg D. The Polycomb complex PRC2 and its mark in life. Nature 2011;469(7330):343–9.

47. Cao R, Wang L, Wang H, et al. Role of histone H3 lysine 27 methylation in Polycomb-group silencing. Science 2002;298(5595):1039–43.

48. Johnson BE, Mazor T, Hong C, et al. Mutational analysis reveals the origin and therapy-driven evolution of recurrent glioma. Science 2014;343(6167):189–93.

49. Wang J, Cazzato E, Ladewig E, et al. Clonal evolution of glioblastoma under therapy. Nat Genet 2016;48(7):768–76.

50. Nassereddine S, Lap CJ, Haroun F, et al. The role of mutant IDH1 and IDH2 inhibitors in the treatment of acute myeloid leukemia. Ann Hematol 2017;96(12):1983–91.

51. Rohle D, Popovici-Muller J, Palaskas N, et al. An inhibitor of mutant IDH1 delays growth and promotes differentiation of glioma cells. Science 2013;340(6132):626–30.

52. Tateishi K, Wakimoto H, Iafrate AJ, et al. Extreme vulnerability of IDH1 mutant cancers to NAD+ depletion. Cancer Cell 2015;28(6):773–84.

53. Turcan S, Makarov V, Taranda J, et al. Mutant-IDH1-dependent chromatin state reprogramming, reversibility, and persistence. Nat Genet 2018;50(1):62–72.

54. Li X, Heyer WD. Homologous recombination in DNA repair and DNA damage tolerance. Cell Res 2008;18(1):99–113.

55. Arnoult N, Correia A, Ma J, et al. Regulation of DNA repair pathway choice in S and G2 phases by the NHEJ inhibitor CYREN. Nature 2017;549(7673):548–52.

56. Chang HHY, Pannunzio NR, Adachi N, et al. Non-homologous DNA end joining and alternative pathways to double-strand break repair. Nat Rev Mol Cell Biol 2017;18(8):495–506.

57. Sulkowski PL, Corso CD, Robinson ND, et al. 2-Hydroxyglutarate produced by neomorphic IDH mutations suppresses homologous recombination and induces PARP inhibitor sensitivity. Sci Transl Med 2017;9(375) [pii:eaal2463].

58. Fong PC, Boss DS, Yap TA, et al. Inhibition of poly(ADP-ribose) polymerase in tumors from BRCA mutation carriers. N Engl J Med 2009;361(2):123–34.

59. Karpel-Massler G, Ishida CT, Bianchetti E, et al. Induction of synthetic lethality in IDH1-mutated gliomas through inhibition of Bcl-xL. Nat Commun 2017;8(1):1067.

60. Delbridge AR, Grabow S, Strasser A, et al. Thirty years of BCL-2: translating cell death discoveries into novel cancer therapies. Nat Rev Cancer 2016;16(2):99–109.

Alterations in the Brain Microenvironment in Diffusely Infiltrating Low-Grade Glioma

Daniela Torres, PhD, Peter Canoll, MD, PhD*

KEYWORDS

- Diffuse astroctyoma • Oligodendroglioma • Microenvironment • Neuronal alterations

KEY POINTS

- Low-grade gliomas, including astrocytomas and oligodendrogliomas, diffusely infiltrate the brain.
- The infiltrating glioma cells intermingle with nonneoplastic brain cells, including astrocytes, microglia, and neurons.
- Many of the clinical symptoms that patients with low-grade gliomas suffer, including epilepsy and neurologic deficits, result from the functional alterations in nonneoplastic brain cells, most notably neurons.
- Molecular and functional alterations of neurons and other nonneoplastic cells in glioma microenvironment remain an understudied problem; however, recently developed experimental tools and models provide new ways to address this important problem.

HISTOPATHOLOGIC/MOLECULAR CLASSIFICATION OF LOW-GRADE GLIOMA, WITH CONTRIBUTIONS FROM THE MICROENVIRONMENT

Diffusely infiltrating gliomas are one of the most common primary brain tumors in adults.[1,2] These types of brain tumors are subclassified based on histologic and molecular features to predict prognosis and guide treatment options.[3,4] However, the unifying histologic feature is that neoplastic cells infiltrate the surrounding brain tissue at the margins of the tumor where they intermingle with nonneoplastic brain cells. Standard of care for patients with glioma includes surgical resection, followed by chemotherapy and radiotherapy.[5–7] However, because these tumors diffusely infiltrate the brain, complete surgical resection is often not possible and the remaining tumor cells eventually result in recurrence. According to the current World Health Organization (WHO) classification system, diffusely infiltrating gliomas are subclassified into astrocytoma or oligodendroglioma on the basis of histologic features and specific molecular alterations (**Fig. 1**). Histologic assessment of glioma tissue analyzes the degree of nuclear atypia, mitotic activity, vascular proliferation, and necrosis, as well as the astrocytic and oligodendroglial features and the patterns of infiltration. Diffusely infiltrating low-grade gliomas (LGG), which include WHO grade II astrocytomas and oligodendrogliomas, typically show a moderate degree of cellular atypia and low mitotic activity, and, by definition, do not have robust vascular proliferation or necrosis. Notably, the majority of diffuse astrocytomas, and virtually all oligodendrogliomas, harbor

Disclosure Statement: Dr Canoll is supported by NIH/NINDS grant numbers R01NS103473, R01NS073610, R01NS052738 and R03NS103125. Dr Torres is supported by NIH/NCI grant number F31CA200375.
Department of Pathology and Cell Biology, Columbia University, Columbia University Medical Center, Irving Cancer Research Center, Room 1002, 1130 St Nicholas Avenue, New York, NY 10032, USA
* Corresponding author.
E-mail address: pc561@cumc.columbia.edu

neurosurgery.theclinics.com

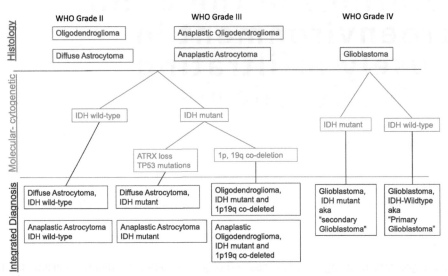

Fig. 1. The integrated histopathologic and molecular World Health Organization (WHO) classification system for diffusely infiltrating gliomas. IDH, isocitrate dehydrogenase.

mutations in the catalytic domain of the metabolic enzyme isocitrate dehydrogenase (IDH), and IDH mutations are now used as a key diagnostic marker that distinguishes the less aggressive IDH1-mutated astrocytoma and oligodendroglioma from the less common but more aggressive IDH-wildtype diffuse astrocytoma. IDH-mutated astrocytomas are further characterized by ATRX loss and TP53 mutations, whereas oligodendrogliomas harbor IDH mutations in combination with codeletions of chromosomes 1p and 19q. Although IDH-mutant gliomas eventually progress to high-grade gliomas (HGG), which include anaplastic oligodendroglioma (WHO grade III), anaplastic astrocytoma (WHO grade III), and glioblastoma (WHO grade IV), this process occurs significantly faster in IDH-wildtype gliomas and, therefore, the molecular classification according to IDH1 status has important diagnostic and prognostic significance.

In addition to its important role in subclassifying diffuse gliomas, mutant IDH1 provides a useful marker for definitively identifying infiltrating glioma cells. Because the IDH mutations are acquired at an early stage in gliomagenesis and are propagated in a clonal fashion, virtually all tumor cells harbor the mutation. In particular, immunohistochemical analysis for the IDH1-R132H mutation, which accounts for approximately 90% of all IDH mutations seen in diffuse gliomas, provides a way to specifically label infiltrating glioma cells and is now used as a standard part of the neuropathologic workup for diffuse gliomas. Immunostains for IDH1-R132H also provide a way to distinguish neoplastic glia from non-neoplastic/reactive glia and highlight the patterns of glioma infiltration into the surrounding brain tissue.[8,9] IDH1 immunostaining thus offers a unique tool for characterizing the cellular composition within the complex microenvironment of diffusely infiltrating gliomas.

Molecular characterization of gliomas by transcriptional analysis using microarrays and RNA-seq has led to the identification of distinct gene expression profiles, including proneural, mesenchymal, neural, and classical subtypes.[10–14] The majority of LGG, including virtually all gliomas that harbor IDH mutations, show a proneural expression pattern characterized by oligodendrocyte lineage genes such as Olig2 and PDGFRα.[8,14,15] Several studies have also revealed a remarkable degree of cellular heterogeneity in gliomas and different biopsies from the same patient can show different expression profiles, demonstrating that the molecular subtype depends on the cellular composition of the tissue sampled.[16–18] Furthermore, the expression profiles of diffusely infiltrating gliomas, as determined by bulk RNA-seq of glioma tissue, is profoundly affected by the contribution of nonneoplastic cells in the brain tumor microenvironment.[16,19] Tissue from the infiltrative margins contains a mixture of glioma cells and nonneoplastic cells, including microglia, astrocytes, oligodendrocytes, and neurons. Identifying the molecular and cellular alterations at the infiltrative margins is of great clinical importance because this tissue is what gets left behind after surgery and will eventually give rise to tumor recurrence. Furthermore, the infiltrative margins of glioma represent the structural and functional interface between neoplastic and nonneoplastic brain tissue that underlies neurologic alterations associated with glioma.

PATIENTS WITH DIFFUSELY INFILTRATING GLIOMA HAVE NEUROLOGIC DEFICITS THAT REVEAL FUNCTIONAL ALTERATIONS IN THE INFILTRATED CORTEX AND SURROUNDING BRAIN TISSUE

Symptoms before a glioma diagnosis include headaches, seizures, and cognitive deficits.[20–23] After diagnosis, patients continue to present with these symptoms, which generally get worse as a result of tumor growth and progression, resulting in a poor quality of life. Neurologic symptoms include impaired working memory, decision making, verbal fluency, and social cognition. Seizures and impaired neurologic function are particularly debilitating in patients with LGG, because patients have a longer survival range and the seizures are often refractory to antiepileptic drugs.[24]

Diffusely infiltrating gliomas can occur anywhere in the central nervous system, but are most commonly localized to the cerebral cortex (frontal and temporal lobes), which explains the impairment in executive function, memory, emotion, or concentration. Worsening of seizures and cognitive function is usually a sign of tumor progression, which is attributed to the diffuse infiltration of tumor cells into functionally important brain regions.[25] However, very little is known about how infiltrating glioma cells affect cortical function and virtually nothing is known about the phenotypic or functional alterations in nonneoplastic cells in diffusely infiltrating glioma.

Notably, patients with LGG often have a presymptomatic period when glioma growth is taking place with no observable symptoms. In fact, gliomas can occupy a remarkably large volume of brain before they manifest clinical symptoms. This property could be explained by reactive adaptions that enable the preservation of neural function despite glioma cell infiltration. This process, which is more generally referred to as reactive plasticity, is considered a response mechanism by which the brain adapts to pathologic stimuli, resulting in the reorganization of neural circuits to preserve remaining function.[26] This concept has been studied in various neurologic diseases, including traumatic brain injury and stroke, and is more recently being explored in low grade glioma.[27] Reactive plasticity in glioma has been studied primarily from a clinical perspective using intraoperative direct electrocortical stimulation.[26] These methods can be used to map cortical brain regions responsible for specific functions such as speech or movement (the so-called eloquent cortex). During subsequent surgical resections, direct electrocortical stimulation has revealed that the same brain region once responsible for a specific function is no longer critical for that function, providing compelling clinical evidence that reactive plasticity is continuously taking place in glioma infiltrated cortex.[28] However, the cellular and molecular mechanisms underlying plasticity associated with LGG are less well-understood. Future studies that address reactive plasticity in LGG could provide important new insight into this phenomenon and the way brain tissue responds to other types of injury and disease.

CURRENT RESEARCH ON NONNEOPLASTIC CELLS FOUND IN GLIOMA BRAIN TISSUE

There is increasing evidence that nonneoplastic cells in the brain tumor microenvironment are key players in the neurologic symptoms in glioma, such as seizures and cognitive dysfunctions, and can contribute to glioma progression and response to treatment. This finding has motivated research on neurons, microglia, astrocytes, and endothelial cells; however, most of the research to date has focused on HGG and the alterations in nonneoplastic cells in the microenvironment of LGG remains an understudied problem.

Resident microglia and monocytes that are derived from the blood are recruited into the brain tumor microenvironment and can contribute to glioma growth and progression in a number of ways. Activated microglia can produce paracrine factors and chemokines that stimulate tumor cell growth and migration.[29–31] Conversely, glioma cells can stimulate microglial motility and activation at the margins of the tumor,[32] suggesting that reciprocal interactions between glioma cells and microglia play an important role in the facilitating glioma invasion into surrounding brain tissue. Several studies have also revealed distinct subpopulations of tumor-associated macrophages, which includes resident microglia and recruited macrophages from the periphery. A recent study used single cell RNA sequencing to show that resident microglia and recruited macrophages have different gene expression signatures and that the expression of blood-derived tumor-associated macrophage markers correlates with poor survival in LGG.[33] These studies also show that IDH mutated astrocytomas and oligodendrogliomas differ with respect to the gene expression signatures derived from the tumor microenvironment, with astrocytomas showing a greater enrichment of microglia/macrophage gene expression and oligodendrogliomas showing a greater enrichment of neuron-specific genes.[19] Notably, there is a shift in the inflammatory microenvironment during glioma progression, with LGG having more resident microglia infiltration compared with HGG, which have more blood-derived tumor-associated macrophages infiltration.[19] Furthermore, studies have shown that these changes in the inflammatory microenvironment may play an important role in glioma progression and modulation of the immune response.[34–36]

Astrocytes are one of the most abundant cells in the brain and they are major component of the neuropathologic response to brain injury or neurologic disease.[37] As a result of injury or disease, astrocytes become reactive, meaning their morphology is altered and they can proliferate around the site of injury.[38] Reactive astrocytes also express a variety of cytokines and growth factors that can stimulate glioma growth and progression.[39] Perivascular astrocytes are also a key component of the blood–brain barrier, and disruptions in the structure and function of astrocyte–vascular interactions, such as displacement of perivascular astrocyte endfeet, may contribute to alterations in vascular permeability and vascular reactivity that is seen in glioma.[40] Notably, a recent study showed that the alterations in vascular reactivity, as seen by blood oxygen level–dependent functional MRI, are more widespread in IDH-wildtype gliomas compared with IDH1-mutated gliomas, suggesting that IDH1 status is a key determinant of vascular function in the infiltrative margins of glioma.[41] These studies also show that alterations in vascular reactivity occur at relatively early stages of glioma progression, and precede the robust "glomeruloid-type" vascular proliferation and alteration in vascular permeability that is seen in HGG. The expression of vascular cell markers also differs significantly between LGG and HGG.[42] Vascular proliferation plays a critical role during the progression from LGG to HGG, during which hypoxia stimulates the expression of cytokines and growth factors that stimulate vascular proliferation and promote growth and invasiveness of glioma cells.[43]

Much of the research on neuronal alterations within glioma has focused on the effects of excess glutamate on neurotoxicity and seizure induction.[44,45] Tumor cells release excess glutamate that binds NMDA receptors and induces an influx of calcium in neurons that results in cell death.[46] High glutamate levels have also been attributed to seizure induction, because seizures are generally characterized by an imbalance of excitatory and inhibitory transmission.[47,48] Glioma cells can express high levels of SLC7A11, a glutamate–cystine exchanger that is responsible for the excess glutamate release from glioma cells, which contributes to glioma-induced seizures and excitotoxicity.[47,49] The effects of neuronal activity on glial progenitors has been explored through optogenetic approaches, which showed that neuronal activation can induce glial progenitor cell proliferation, suggesting that neuronal activity may contribute to glioma cell proliferation.[50–52] Further characterization of the effects of glioma cells on neurons is essential because this effect may underlie the neurologic symptoms associated with glioma and can provide therapeutic alternatives for these symptoms.

METHODS USED TO CHARACTERIZE NONNEOPLASTIC CELLS IN DIFFUSELY INFILTRATING GLIOMA: CHALLENGES AND OPPORTUNITIES

Neuropathologists and researchers have historically used immunohistochemical analysis to identify alterations the molecular and cellular composition of brain tumors. Although there are a few markers, such as IDH1-R132H, which provide selective staining of specific glioma-associated mutated alleles, immunohistochemical stains can also be used to highlight alterations in different cellular components of the tumor microenvironment, such as microglia, astrocytes, and neurons (**Fig. 2**). In situ hybridization has also been used to identify cell type specific alterations in RNA levels from brain tumor tissue; however,

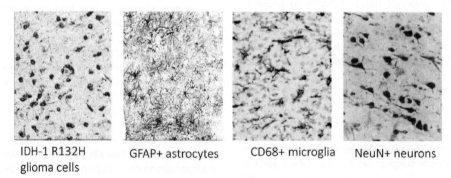

IDH-1 R132H glioma cells   GFAP+ astrocytes   CD68+ microglia   NeuN+ neurons

Fig. 2. Immunohistochemical stains label different cell types at the infiltrative margins of glioma. IDH, isocitrate dehydrogenase (H&E, original magnification ×20).

most of these studies have been limited to identifying alterations in just 1 transcript per tissue section. The development of highly multiplexed techniques, such as Seq-FISH,[53] now allows for profiling the expression of hundreds of transcripts at the single cell level in histologic sections of brain tissue and the application of such techniques to glioma tissue offers a powerful way to characterize the transcriptional alterations across multiple cell types in the brain tumor microenvironment.

Next-generation sequencing has provided a genome-wide readout of molecular alterations in glioma tissue. The majority of studies have analyzed RNA and DNA isolated from homogenized tissue samples that contain all the different cell types in the glioma microenvironment. Thus, the data represent a composite of signatures that makes it difficult to identify alterations in specific subpopulations of cells. Furthermore, variations in the relative abundance of different cell types can have marked effects on the composite signature, which further confound the interpretation of the data. One approach to address the challenge of complex cellular composition of brain tumors has been to implement computational algorithms that can deconvolve cell-type–specific expression signatures from bulk RNA-seq data based on lineage-specific markers.[16,54] One major advantage of this approach is that it provides information on cell-type–specific expression patterns within the context of the intact tumor microenvironment.

Single cell RNA-seq provides another approach to identifying cell-type–specific alterations and has been has been applied to glioma tissue in a number of recent studies.[17,19,33,55,56] These studies have provided important new insights in the cellular heterogeneity observed between and within different gliomas and have characterized alterations, both in neoplastic and nonneoplastic cells within glioma microenvironment. However, current methods of single cell RNA-seq require that that individual cells are isolated from tissue through a process of enzymatic digestion and mechanical isolation. There are multiple caveats associated with these methods that should be considered when assessing results from this area of research including, (1) enzymatic and physical dissociation induces stress that can influence gene expression, (2) gene expression from cell types that are less abundant, or harder to isolate, in the tissue may not be well-represented, and (3) microdissection and enzymatic dissociation can damage cell processes and deplete transcripts which are localized to these compartments.[57] Cells with elaborate cytoplasmic processes, such as neurons, are particularly subject to this

constraint because their cellular processes are prone to damage during dissociation of the tissue. These technical challenges have limited the molecular profiling of specific nonneoplastic cell types, such as neurons, which reside in the glioma microenvironment.

Mouse models can also provide an experimental system in which to study the brain tumor microenvironment. There are several different transgenic mouse models that recapitulate the key histopathologic and molecular features of human glioma.[54,58–63] Notably, many of these models begin as LGG that diffusely infiltrate the brain and then, over the course of weeks or months, progress to HGG. These mouse models also develop seizures during gliomagenesis, which recapitulates the neurologic dysfunction seen in patients with glioma. Notably, these mouse models can be genetically engineered to express cell-type–specific reporters, such as the bacTRAP and RiboTag systems that allow transcriptional and translational profiling of distinct cell types within the brain tumor microenvironment.[54,64–67] These mouse models offer the potential to characterize molecular alterations in a variety of different cell types at different stages of glioma progression and to test the effects of molecular and pharmacologic perturbations in well-controlled preclinical experiments.

SUMMARY

The studies referenced in this review highlight the importance of the brain tumor microenvironment in glioma. Although most research to date has focused on nonneoplastic cell alterations in HGG, it is essential to identify nonneoplastic cell alterations in LGG in which glioma cells diffusely invade surrounding brain tissue and are closely intermingled with nonneoplastic cells types. Recent research suggests that targeting nonneoplastic cell types can be a potential therapy to treat glioma growth. For example, there is the possibility that one might also affect glioma growth by targeting neuronal activity. Studying the alterations in nonneoplastic cell types in glioma may also give new insights into the way brain tissue responds to injury and, by better understanding the tissue response, we may gain new insights into the mechanisms of reactive plasticity. Recently developed experimental methods now make it possible to dissect the complex cellular alterations in brain tissue, which can be applied to identifying the alterations in nonneoplastic cell types in the brain tumor microenvironment. Low-grade diffusely infiltrating gliomas provide a unique and important disease system to study the complex cellular alterations that contribute to tumor growth and neurologic symptoms seen in patients with gliomas.

REFERENCES

1. Ostrom QT, Gittleman H, Liao P, et al. CBTRUS Statistical Report: primary brain and other central nervous system tumors diagnosed in the United States in 2010-2014. Neuro Oncol 2017;19(suppl_5):v1–88.
2. Weller M, Wick W, Aldape K, et al. Glioma. Nat Rev Dis Primers 2015;1:15017.
3. Masui K, Mischel PS, Reifenberger G. Chapter 6 - molecular classification of gliomas. In: Berger MS, Weller M, editors. Handbook of clinical neurology, vol. 134. Amsterdam (Netherlands): Elsevier; 2016. p. 97–120.
4. Louis DN, Perry A, Reifenberger G, et al. The 2016 World Health Organization classification of tumors of the central nervous system: a summary. Acta Neuropathol 2016;131(6):803–20.
5. Davis ME. Glioblastoma: overview of disease and treatment. Clin J Oncol Nurs 2016;20(5):S2–8.
6. van den Bent MJ, Snijders TJ, Bromberg JEC. Current treatment of low grade gliomas. Memo 2012; 5(3):223–7.
7. Stupp R, Mason WP, van den Bent MJ, et al. Radiotherapy plus concomitant and adjuvant temozolomide for glioblastoma. N Engl J Med 2005;352(10): 987–96.
8. Tsankova NM, Canoll P. Advances in genetic and epigenetic analyses of gliomas: a neuropathological perspective. J Neurooncol 2014;119(3):481–90.
9. Zetterling M, Roodakker KR, Berntsson SG, et al. Extension of diffuse low-grade gliomas beyond radiological borders as shown by the coregistration of histopathological and magnetic resonance imaging data. J Neurosurg 2016;125(5):1155–66.
10. Verhaak RG, Hoadley KA, Purdom E, et al. Integrated genomic analysis identifies clinically relevant subtypes of glioblastoma characterized by abnormalities in PDGFRA, IDH1, EGFR, and NF1. Cancer Cell 2010;17(1):98–110.
11. Brennan CW, Verhaak RG, McKenna A, et al. The somatic genomic landscape of glioblastoma. Cell 2013;155(2):462–77.
12. Phillips HS, Kharbanda S, Chen R, et al. Molecular subclasses of high-grade glioma predict prognosis, delineate a pattern of disease progression, and resemble stages in neurogenesis. Cancer Cell 2006;9(3):157–73.
13. Parsons DW, Jones S, Zhang X, et al. An integrated genomic analysis of human glioblastoma multiforme. Science 2008;321(5897):1807.
14. Zong H, Verhaak RG, Canoll P. The cellular origin for malignant glioma and prospects for clinical advancements. Expert Rev Mol Diagn 2012;12(4): 383–94.
15. Cooper LA, Gutman DA, Long Q, et al. The proneural molecular signature is enriched in oligodendrogliomas and predicts improved survival among diffuse gliomas. PLoS One 2010;5(9):e12548.
16. Gill BJ, Pisapia DJ, Malone HR, et al. MRI-localized biopsies reveal subtype-specific differences in molecular and cellular composition at the margins of glioblastoma. Proc Natl Acad Sci U S A 2014; 111(34):12550–5.
17. Patel AP, Tirosh I, Trombetta JJ, et al. Single-cell RNA-seq highlights intratumoral heterogeneity in primary glioblastoma. Science 2014;344(6190): 1396–401.
18. Sottoriva A, Spiteri I, Piccirillo SG, et al. Intratumor heterogeneity in human glioblastoma reflects cancer evolutionary dynamics. Proc Natl Acad Sci U S A 2013;110(10):4009–14.
19. Venteicher AS, Tirosh I, Hebert C, et al. Decoupling genetics, lineages, and microenvironment in IDH-mutant gliomas by single-cell RNA-seq. Science 2017;355(6332) [pii:eaai8478].
20. Taphoorn MJB, Klein M. Cognitive deficits in adult patients with brain tumours. Lancet Neurol 2004; 3(3):159–68.
21. Bosma I, Vos MJ, Heimans JJ, et al. The course of neurocognitive functioning in high-grade glioma patients. Neuro Oncol 2007;9(1):53–62.
22. Miotto EC, Silva Junior A, Silva CC, et al. Cognitive impairments in patients with low grade gliomas and high grade gliomas. Arq Neuropsiquiatr 2011; 69:596–601.
23. Bergo E, Lombardi G, Pambuku A, et al. Cognitive rehabilitation in patients with gliomas and other brain tumors: state of the art. Biomed Res Int 2016;2016:11.
24. Vecht CJ, Kerkhof M, Duran-Pena A. Seizure prognosis in brain tumors: new insights and evidence-based management. Oncologist 2014;19(7):751–9.
25. Bergo E, Lombardi G, Guglieri I, et al. Neurocognitive functions and health-related quality of life in glioblastoma patients: a concise review of the literature. Eur J Cancer Care (Engl) 2015. [Epub ahead of print].
26. Kong NW, Gibb WR, Tate MC. Neuroplasticity: insights from patients harboring gliomas. Neural Plast 2016;2016:12.
27. Desmurget M, Bonnetblanc F, Duffau H. Contrasting acute and slow-growing lesions: a new door to brain plasticity. Brain 2007;130(4):898–914.
28. Duffau H. Diffuse low-grade gliomas and neuroplasticity. Diagn Interv Imaging 2014;95(10):945–55.
29. Hambardzumyan D, Gutmann DH, Kettenmann H. The role of microglia and macrophages in glioma maintenance and progression. Nat Neurosci 2015; 19:20.

30. Wei J, Gabrusiewicz K, Heimberger A. The controversial role of microglia in malignant gliomas. Clin Dev Immunol 2013;2013:12.

31. Coniglio SJ, Segall JE. Review: molecular mechanism of microglia stimulated glioblastoma invasion. Matrix Biol 2013;32(7):372–80.

32. Juliano J, Gil O, Hawkins-Daarud A, et al. Comparative dynamics of microglial and glioma cell motility at the infiltrative margin of brain tumours. J R Soc Interface 2018;15(139) [pii:20170582].

33. Muller S, Kohanbash G, Liu SJ, et al. Single-cell profiling of human gliomas reveals macrophage ontogeny as a basis for regional differences in macrophage activation in the tumor microenvironment. Genome Biol 2017;18(1):234.

34. Rajappa P, Cobb WS, Vartanian E, et al. Malignant astrocytic tumor progression potentiated by JAK-mediated recruitment of myeloid cells. Clin Cancer Res 2017;23(12):3109–19.

35. Huang Y, Rajappa P, Hu W, et al. A proangiogenic signaling axis in myeloid cells promotes malignant progression of glioma. J Clin Invest 2017;127(5):1826–38.

36. Ha ET, Antonios JP, Soto H, et al. Chronic inflammation drives glioma growth: cellular and molecular factors responsible for an immunosuppressive microenvironment. Neuroimmunology and Neuroinflammation 2014;1(2):66–76.

37. Liddelow SA, Barres BA. Reactive astrocytes: production, function, and therapeutic potential. Immunity 2017;46(6):957–67.

38. Buffo A, Rite I, Tripathi P, et al. Origin and progeny of reactive gliosis: a source of multipotent cells in the injured brain. Proc Natl Acad Sci U S A 2008;105(9):3581–6.

39. Guan X, Hasan MN, Maniar S, et al. Reactive astrocytes in glioblastoma multiforme. Mol Neurobiol 2018;55(8):6927–38.

40. Chow DS, Horenstein CI, Canoll P, et al. Glioblastoma induces vascular dysregulation in nonenhancing peritumoral regions in humans. AJR Am J Roentgenol 2016;206(5):1073–81.

41. Englander ZK, Horenstein CI, Bowden SG, et al. Extent of BOLD vascular dysregulation is greater in diffuse gliomas without isocitrate dehydrogenase 1 R132H mutation. Radiology 2018;287(3):965–72.

42. Miebach S, Grau S, Hummel V, et al. Isolation and culture of microvascular endothelial cells from gliomas of different WHO grades. J Neurooncol 2006;76(1):39–48.

43. Xu R, Pisapia D, Greenfield JP. Malignant transformation in glioma steered by an angiogenic switch: defining a role for bone marrow-derived cells. Cureus 2016;8(1):e471.

44. Huberfeld G, Vecht CJ. Seizures and gliomas—towards a single therapeutic approach. Nat Rev Neurol 2016;12(4):204–16.

45. de Groot J, Sontheimer H. Glutamate and the biology of gliomas. Glia 2011;59(8):1181–9.

46. Sontheimer H. A role for glutamate in growth and invasion of primary brain tumors. J Neurochem 2008;105(2):287–95.

47. Buckingham SC, Campbell SL, Haas BR, et al. Glutamate release by primary brain tumors induces epileptic activity. Nat Med 2011;17(10):1269–74.

48. Campbell SL, Buckingham SC, Sontheimer H. Human glioma cells induce hyperexcitability in cortical networks. Epilepsia 2012;53(8):1360–70.

49. Sørensen MF, Heimisdóttir SB, Sørensen MD, et al. High expression of cystine–glutamate antiporter xCT (SLC7A11) is an independent biomarker for epileptic seizures at diagnosis in glioma. J Neurooncol 2018;138(1):49–53.

50. Venkatesh Humsa S, Johung Tessa B, Caretti V, et al. Neuronal activity promotes glioma growth through neuroligin-3 secretion. Cell 2015;161(4):803–16.

51. Gillespie S, Monje M. An active role for neurons in glioma progression: making sense of Scherer's structures. Neuro Oncol 2018;20(10):1292–9.

52. Venkatesh HS, Tam LT, Woo PJ, et al. Targeting neuronal activity-regulated neuroligin-3 dependency in high-grade glioma. Nature 2017;549(7673):533–7.

53. Shah S, Lubeck E, Zhou W, et al. seqFISH accurately detects transcripts in single cells and reveals robust spatial organization in the hippocampus. Neuron 2017;94(4):752–758 e751.

54. Gonzalez C, Sims JS, Hornstein N, et al. Ribosome profiling reveals a cell-type-specific translational landscape in brain tumors. J Neurosci 2014;34(33):10924–36.

55. Tirosh I, Suvà ML. Dissecting human gliomas by single-cell RNA sequencing. Neuro Oncol 2018;20(1):37–43.

56. Darmanis S, Sloan SA, Croote D, et al. Single-cell RNA-seq analysis of infiltrating neoplastic cells at the migrating front of human glioblastoma. Cell Rep 2017;21(5):1399–410.

57. Poulin J-F, Tasic B, Hjerling-Leffler J, et al. Disentangling neural cell diversity using single-cell transcriptomics. Nat Neurosci 2016;19:1131–41.

58. Dai C, Celestino JC, Okada Y, et al. PDGF autocrine stimulation dedifferentiates cultured astrocytes and induces oligodendrogliomas and oligoastrocytomas from neural progenitors and astrocytes in vivo. Genes Dev 2001;15(15):1913–25.

59. Weiss WA, Burns MJ, Hackett C, et al. Genetic determinants of malignancy in a mouse model for oligodendroglioma. Cancer Res 2003;63(7):1589–95.

60. Lei L, Sonabend AM, Guarnieri P, et al. Glioblastoma models reveal the connection between adult glial progenitors and the proneural phenotype. PLoS One 2011;6(5):e20041.

61. Liu C, Sage JC, Miller MR, et al. Mosaic analysis with double markers reveals tumor cell of origin in glioma. Cell 2011;146(2):209–21.

62. Sonabend AM, Bansal M, Guarnieri P, et al. The transcriptional regulatory network of proneural glioma determines the genetic alterations selected during tumor progression. Cancer Res 2014;74(5): 1440–51.

63. Herting CJ, Chen Z, Pitter KL, et al. Genetic driver mutations define the expression signature and microenvironmental composition of high-grade gliomas. Glia 2017;65(12):1914–26.

64. Dougherty JD, Schmidt EF, Nakajima M, et al. Analytical approaches to RNA profiling data for the identification of genes enriched in specific cells. Nucleic Acids Res 2010;38(13):4218–30.

65. Sanz E, Yang L, Su T, et al. Cell-type-specific isolation of ribosome-associated mRNA from complex tissues. Proc Natl Acad Sci U S A 2009;106(33): 13939–44.

66. Dougherty JD, Fomchenko EI, Akuffo AA, et al. Candidate pathways for promoting differentiation or quiescence of oligodendrocyte progenitor-like cells in glioma. Cancer Res 2012;72(18):4856–68.

67. Hornstein N, Torres D, Das Sharma S, et al. Ligation-free ribosome profiling of cell type-specific translation in the brain. Genome Biol 2016; 17(1):149.

Clinical and Imaging

Clinical Presentation, Natural History, and Prognosis of Diffuse Low-Grade Gliomas

Anja Smits, MD, PhD[a,b],*, Asgeir S. Jakola, MD, PhD[a,c,d]

KEYWORDS

- Diffuse low-grade gliomas • Symptoms • Natural history • Prognosis

KEY POINTS

- The natural course of diffuse low-grade glioma (DLGG) consists of a silent period when diagnosis is still unknown, followed by a symptomatic period and a subsequent progressive phase.
- Most patients present with new-onset seizures but emotional and/or cognitive symptoms may occur already during the silent phase, indicating that this phase is not equivalent with asymptomatic.
- Prognosis of patients with DLGG is highly variable. Clinical parameters in combination with molecular tumor profiles are used to define prognostic risk groups and to improve individual treatment decisions.

INTRODUCTION

Diffuse low-grade gliomas (DLGGs) are slow-growing primary brain tumors classified as mainly astrocytomas or oligodendrogliomas World Health Organization (WHO) grade II by the WHO classification of brain tumors.[1] DLGGs are characterized by low proliferation but extensive infiltration into the surrounding brain. Large-scale genomic profiling studies have introduced the term "lower-grade gliomas," referring to 3 nonoverlapping molecular subtypes of gliomas WHO grade II and grade IIII with separate clinical outcome.[2] In this article, DLGG refers to gliomas WHO grade II unless otherwise stated.

DLGGs occur as hypointense lesions on T1-weighted images and hyperintense lesions on fluid-attenuated inversion recovery or T2-weighted sequences. Morphologic MRI tends to underestimate the extension of DLGGs and their diffuse infiltrative growth in white matter fibers.[3,4] The absence of contrast enhancement on gadolinium-based MRI is characteristic for DLGGs but with low specificity and sensitivity to differentiate DLGGs from high-grade gliomas. Approximately one-fifth of DLGGs enhance, whereas up to one-third of nonenhancing gliomas are histologic high-grade gliomas.[5]

DLGGs occur in adult life with a peak incidence at approximately 30 to 35 years. Over time, DLGGs show a tendency to transform into high-grade gliomas and will eventually lead to death,[6] but the clinical course of this patient group is surprisingly diverse. Most tumors expand in volume by only a few millimeters per year and patients may remain free from any debilitating symptoms for many

Disclosure: The authors have nothing to disclose.
[a] Institute of Neuroscience and Physiology, Sahlgrenska Academy, Gothenburg, Sweden; [b] Department of Neuroscience, Section of Neurology, Uppsala University, 751 85 Uppsala, Sweden; [c] Department of Neurosurgery, Sahlgrenska University Hospital, Blå Stråket 5, 41345 Gothenburg, Sweden; [d] Department of Neurosurgery, St Olavs Hospital, Prinsesse Kristinas gate 3, 7030 Trondheim, Norway
* Corresponding author. Department of Neuroscience and Physiology, Sahlgrenska University Hospital, Blå Stråket 7, Plan 3, Gothenburg 41345, Sweden.
E-mail address: anja.smits@neuro.uu.se

Neurosurg Clin N Am 30 (2019) 35–42
https://doi.org/10.1016/j.nec.2018.08.002
1042-3680/19/

years.[7] These specific tumor features impose a major challenge on the clinical management, requiring an individualized approach for each patient to decide optimal treatment strategies, as well as optimal timing of treatment. In balancing the pros and cons of tumor treatment and symptomatic treatment, the ability to maintain a satisfactory professional, social, and emotional quality of life needs to be considered. It has become evident that additional measures beyond progression-free and overall survival for this patient group are important in clinical trials.[8] Here we discuss some of the clinical challenges at disease presentation with regard to the natural history of DLGG and the long-term prognosis of patients, illustrated in **Fig. 1**.

CLINICAL PRESENTATION

Over time, the tumor interferes with normal brain function by disrupting functional connectivity of brain networks within peritumoral and distant brain areas, thereby promoting seizure activity.[9] Indeed, in 70% to 90% of all patients with DLGG, new-onset seizures are the presenting symptoms leading to tumor diagnosis. The slow growth of the tumor allows for cortical adaptor mechanisms enabling functional and morphologic reorganization of the brain, and neurologic deficits are usually absent at disease onset.[10] It is well-known though that the plasticity of subcortical structures compared with the cortex is significantly reduced. Patients with tumor infiltration of the subcortical

connectivity are therefore at higher risk to develop tumor-related symptoms at the early phase. The prevalence of functional deficits at presentation in these patients, especially of subtle cognitive deficits, is probably underestimated.[11]

Seizure Semiology

Brain tumor–related seizures are classified as focal seizures or focal to bilateral tonic-clonic seizures.[12] Seizure semiology reflects the specific tumor localization with the somatotopic organization of cortical brain functions. The frontal lobe, as the most common location of DLGGs, is associated with a variety of seizures. Asymmetric tonic seizures with tonic arm extension and elevation, followed by forced head deviation, occur with seizures originating in the supplementary motor area. Jacksonian motor or somatosensory seizures are associated with peri-rolandic areas, whereas speech arrest or motor agitation are seen with deeply seated frontal lobe tumors. Patients with temporal lobe tumors report characteristic symptoms consisting of déjà vu phenomena, visceral sensations, auditory hallucinations, or language and memory disturbances. Insular seizures have been associated with laryngeal discomfort, thoracic and abdominal oppression or dyspnea, and unpleasant paresthesia or warmth sensations in the face and larger cutaneous territory, followed by dysarthria and focal motor convulsions.[13] The occipital region is a less common location for DLGGs. Patients with occipital lobe tumors may

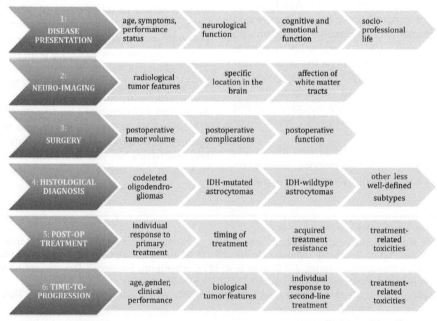

Fig. 1. Illustration of the clinical parameters that affect the natural course and prognosis of patients with DLGG. Post-op, postoperative.

experience positive visual symptoms, but also visual field defects or blurred vision during seizure activity, mimicking migraine headaches.

Cognitive Symptoms

Most of our knowledge on cognitive performance at the time of diagnosis comes from observational studies in which cognitive function and/or language has been evaluated as baseline performance before treatment.[14,15] Impairment of executive functions, attention, concentration, and memory can be attributed to the tumor itself, to poor seizure control, antiepileptic drug treatment, or a combination of these factors.[16] Cognitive deficits are associated with reduced quality of life and need to be identified as early as possible.[17,18] The inclusion of neuropsychological examination as part of the diagnostic procedure at presentation is therefore justified, and the use of common assessment protocols between different centers will contribute to a deeper understanding of cognitive function in DLGG.[19] Still, it should be acknowledged that most patients show performance comparable to the healthy population and enjoy a normal social and professional life at disease presentation. The elderly population of patients with DLGG, however, presents more often with debilitating cognitive impairment and language disorders.[20] The differences in symptoms at disease onset with higher age, favoring neurologic and cognitive deficits over seizures, reflect a generally more aggressive tumor behavior in elderly patients with glioma.

Emotional and Psychological Symptoms

Depression and anxiety are caused by the psychological stress of brain tumor diagnosis and/or by the tumor itself. In general, patients with right-sided primary brain tumors have higher anxiety levels than patients with left-sided tumors,[21] but tumor sidedness does not seem to affect the overall quality of life.[22] Fatigue, including concentration problems and reduced motivation and physical activity, is frequently reported by patients with cancer. The prevalence and severity of fatigue at the time of diagnosis in patients with DLGG remain to be determined. Fatigue in this patient group has been studied mostly with regard to treatment or in long-term survivors, where it was reported as a severe problem for many patients.[23]

Incidental Diffuse Low-Grade Gliomas

Approximately 3% to 10% of all DLGGs are discovered when radiological examination is performed for reasons unrelated to the tumor and considered as incidental DLGG.[24,25] In general, patients with incidental DLGG have smaller tumor volume, less frequent involvement of eloquent areas, and better performance status scores.[24,26] Although incidental in nature, patients may suffer from cognitive symptoms that are not recognized as such before imaging diagnosis.[27] It was reported that 36% of patients with DLGG encountered adjusted work tasks or reduced workload 1 year before tumor diagnosis, which is higher than expected in the healthy working population.[28]

NATURAL HISTORY

The natural course of DLGG consists of a silent period, followed by a symptomatic period and a subsequent progressive phase.

Silent Phase

The question whether patients with incidental DLGG should undergo early tumor resection is closely related to the question of whether incidental DLGGs constitute a specific subpopulation of tumors. As mentioned, a predominance of oligodendroglial tumors has been reported among incidental DLGGs.[24,26] Similar to the discussion for breast cancer, it can be argued if it is good that DLGGs are small or simply if they are small because they are good.[29] However, because incidental DLGGs have growth dynamics similar to symptomatic DLGGs, a completely different clinical course is unlikely.[24,25] Furthermore, a case of acute progressive incidental DLGG with radiological progression preceding clinical deterioration was reported,[30] illustrating the inadequateness of clinical surveillance. It is expected that incidental findings will increase in clinical practice with more liberal use of MRI, although this increase will be larger for benign lesions.[31] Incidental DLGGs will intentionally increase if screening programs are launched.[32]

Symptomatic Phase

A particular challenge for the clinician following radiological diagnosis is the interpretation of clinically stable disease, which for many patients may stretch over several years. From a radiological point of view, there is no such state as stable disease. DLGGs continue to grow also during symptom-free time intervals.[3] The assessment of volumetric growth over time provides prognostic information as well as valuable diagnostic information, when nontumorous lesions or more uncommon intra-axial low-grade tumors are being considered as differential diagnosis. If the largest diameter of the lesion grows with a rate of approximately 4 mm per year, the likelihood increases that it is indeed a DLGG.[33]

Surgery results in cytoreduction but does not affect the subsequent growth rate of DLGG.

Irradiation and chemotherapy, on the other hand, can temporarily slow down the growth curve of the tumor, although there are no long-lasting effects on tumor growth. After an initial decrease in growth rate, most tumors resume their initial growth on discontinuation of temozolomide. The effect on mean tumor diameter was shown to be especially brief in non-codeleted DLGGs, giving support for acquired chemoresistance.[34] Results from growth kinetic studies are consistent with clinical data on patient outcome as reported by the randomized trials of DLGGs. The European Organisation for Research and Treatment of Cancer (EORTC) 22845 trial of the long-term efficacy of early versus delayed radiotherapy showed prolonged progression-free survival but no increased overall survival after early radiotherapy.[35] The EORTC 22033-26033 trial, randomizing high-risk patients to temozolomide or radiotherapy, found no significant differences in progression-free survival between the 2 arms.[36] The health-related quality of life was similar for patients treated with standard radiotherapy or with primary chemotherapy.[37]

Progressive Phase

Because DLGGs show continuous growth during the entire low-grade phase, the term progression with respect to DLGGs can be debated, but the occurrence of malignant transformation clearly represents an important event. Some patients may experience clinical progression before radiological progression, but radiological signs of malignant transformation can precede or occur parallel with clinical progression. For this reason, clinical follow-up of symptoms and signs of disease combined with radiological surveillance at frequent intervals is needed to detect this event. The time to malignant transformation differs considerably between patients and to accurately predict this event for individual patients is one of the main challenges in clinical practice. It is likely that delaying malignant transformation is crucial to improve survival in DLGG. In a recent case series, the yearly incidence of malignant transformation was 0.17 per person per year of follow-up, with transformation closely linked to subsequent death.[6] Risk factors for transformation included older age, male sex, multiple tumor locations, the use of chemotherapy alone, and the presence of residual disease, whereas the impact of tumor size and molecular tumor status could not be evaluated in this study.[6]

Altering the Natural History

Extensive cytoreductive surgery with removal of microscopic anaplastic foci may delay malignant transformation,[38,39] thereby altering the natural history of the disease. It is likely that a delay in malignant transformation can also be obtained by combined radiotherapy and chemotherapy, based on the results from the Radiation Therapy Oncology Group 9202 trial, in which patients were randomly selected to radiotherapy alone or to radiotherapy followed by 6 cycles of PCV (Procarbazine, CCNU, and Vincristine).[40] There was extensive crossover in the radiotherapy group, with 77% of included patients receiving salvage chemotherapy, presumably after transformation occurred, but at this time point chemotherapy did not result in a similar clinical effect.[41] Therapy may, on the other hand, also negatively affect the natural history. Temozolomide was shown to induce a hypermutation phenotype in a subset of patients with DLGG, resulting in acquired resistance to temozolomide.[42]

PROGNOSIS

The concept that prognostic subtypes of DLGG are tightly associated with molecular signaling pathways has dramatically altered our understanding of glioma biology. Molecular tumor markers have been established as important predictors of biology and patient outcome.[43] Despite the huge scientific impact of these discoveries, the clinical benefits in terms of patient outcome are still limited. In spite of optimal management by surgery, radiotherapy, and chemotherapy, even the prognostic most favorable subgroup of isocitrate dehydrogenase (IDH)-mutant 1p19q codeleted oligodendrogliomas, will eventually transform into malignant gliomas. The 5-year overall and progression-free survival rates of DLGG in randomized studies range from, respectively, 58% to 72% and 37% to 55%.[44] One of the major obstacles for improvement of survival is the lack of effective biologically based treatment for DLGG. Current standard therapy comprises only PCV and temozolomide, and new targeted treatment strategies for DLGG are highly warranted. One interesting option that is currently tested for lower-grade gliomas is direct inhibition of the IDH mutant enzyme.[45] Mutation of the IDH gene is an early event in gliomagenesis that is retained after malignant transformation.[46]

Tumor Heterogeneity

Targeted drug therapy has been tested for patients with glioblastomas, but so far with disappointing results. The modest effect in these tumors has been contributed to resistance mechanisms, the poor blood-brain barrier penetration, the redundancy of signaling pathways offering escape mechanisms, and to tumor heterogeneity.[45] Molecular heterogeneity is not unique for glioblastomas, but is seen also in DLGGs, even within histologic entities defined by IDH mutations and 1p19q codeletions. An overview of the studies illustrating the molecular heterogeneity in DLGGs is beyond the scope of this review. Instead, we discuss some of the patient-related and tumor-related factors behind the clinical heterogeneity of DLGGs.

Clinical Heterogeneity

As mentioned, DLGG as a disease entity is characterized by a large clinical heterogeneity. Prognostic models have been used based on the presence of clinical prognostic factors, in which the total number of unfavorable parameters determines the prognostic score for individual patients. **Table 1** summarizes some of the main findings from these studies. The preoperative classification

model introduced by the University of California, San Francisco-Group, included tumor location in eloquent areas, Karnofsky performance scale score, and maximum tumor diameter as prognostic variables.[47] Pooled analysis of patients enrolled in the EORTC trials 22844 and 22845 identified astrocytoma histology, age ≥40, the presence of neurologic deficits, tumor diameter ≥6 cm, and tumor crossing the midline as prognostic factors for survival.[48] A validated prognostic score was presented later after central pathology review, identifying patients with low, intermediate, and high risk based on the presence of baseline neurologic deficits, less than 30 weeks since first symptoms, astrocytic tumor type, and tumor diameter greater than 5 cm.[49] Several studies have confirmed the prognostic value of single parameters, such as the impact of cognitive deficits or seizures at onset,[50,51] or identified new parameters for DLGG, such as the type of contrast enhancement, the tumor growth rate, and the

Table 1
Overview of studies that have identified important clinical prognostic factors for patients with diffuse low-grade glioma

Prognostic Factors	Favorable	Unfavorable	Comments	References
Strongest prognostic impact				
Age	High	Low	Cutoff at 40 y	Pignatti et al,[48] 2002
			Cutoff at 50 y	Chang et al,[47] 2008
Histology	Oligodendroglioma	Astrocytoma	Assoc with mol profile	Pignatti et al,[48] 2002; Gorlia et al,[49] 2013
IDH mutation status	Mutated	Wild type		Brat et al,[2] 2015
1p19q chromosome	Codeleted	Intact		Brat et al,[2] 2015
Additional prognostic factors				
Volume growth	≤ 4 mm/y	> 4 mm/y	Assoc with histology	Pallud et al,[52] 2013
Time since first symptoms	< 30 wk	≥ 30 wk		Gorlia et al,[49] 2013
Diameter size	Small	Large	Cutoff at 6 cm	Pignatti et al,[48] 2002
			Cutoff at 4 cm	Chang et al,[47] 2008
			Cutoff at 5 cm	Gorlia et al,[49] 2013
Contrast enhancement	No CE	CE present	Nodular type of CE	Pallud et al,[53] 2009
Tumor location	Frontal	Crossing midline	Assoc with mol profile	Capelle et al,[54] 2013
Performance status	KPS > 80	KPS ≤ 80		Chang et al,[47] 2008
Seizures vs neurological deficits	Yes vs no	No vs yes		Pignatti et al,[48] 2002; Pallud et al,[51] 2014
Cognitive deficits	MMSE > 26	MMSE ≤ 26		Daniels et al,[50] 2011
Functional area		Eloquent area	Assoc with ER	Chang et al,[47] 2008

Abbreviations: Assoc, associated; CE, contrast enhancement; ER, extent of resection; KPS, Karnofsky performance scale; MMSE, mini-mental status examination; Mol, molecular.

specific tumor location.[52–54] The value of combining clinical parameters with molecular tumor markers is now beginning to emerge to better understand the heterogeneity of DLGGs. Some examples are the established interactions between the molecular tumor profile with tumor location or the radiological tumor features.[55,56]

SUMMARY

Most patients with DLGG present with seizures and have no significant disability at disease onset. Although the prognosis and the natural course of individual patients show a large diversity, the mean survival in this patient group is significantly impaired due to malignant tumor transformation that occurs in an unpredictable manner. Prognosis at group-level is strongly associated with molecular tumor profile but varies also within histologic tumor entities defined by IDH gene mutations and codeletions at chromosome 1p/19q. The clinical heterogeneity of DLGG is exemplified by the strong prognostic impact of multiple clinical parameters at disease onset that have been validated by large randomized trials. Future challenges need to take advantage of new and fast technologies for molecular screening of the tumor, in combination with individualized treatment and care of patients.

REFERENCES

1. Louis DN, Perry A, Reifenberger G, et al. The 2016 World Health Organization classification of tumors of the central nervous system: a summary. Acta Neuropathol 2016;131(6):803–20.
2. Brat DJ, Verhaak RG, Aldape KD, et al. Comprehensive, integrative genomic analysis of diffuse lower-grade gliomas. N Engl J Med 2015;372(26): 2481–98.
3. Pallud J, Varlet P, Devaux B, et al. Diffuse low-grade oligodendrogliomas extend beyond MRI-defined abnormalities. Neurology 2010;74(21): 1724–31.
4. Zetterling M, Roodakker KR, Berntsson SG, et al. Extension of diffuse low-grade gliomas beyond radiological borders as shown by the coregistration of histopathological and magnetic resonance imaging data. J Neurosurg 2016;125(5):1155–66.
5. Scott JN, Brasher PM, Sevick RJ, et al. How often are nonenhancing supratentorial gliomas malignant? A population study. Neurology 2002;59(6):947–9.
6. Murphy ES, Leyrer CM, Parsons M, et al. Risk factors for malignant transformation of low-grade glioma. Int J Radiat Oncol Biol Phys 2018;100(4): 965–71.
7. Mandonnet E, Delattre J-YY, Tanguy M-LL, et al. Continuous growth of mean tumor diameter in a subset of grade II gliomas. Ann Neurol 2003;53(4): 524–8.
8. Avila EK, Chamberlain M, Schiff D, et al. Seizure control as a new metric in assessing efficacy of tumor treatment in low-grade glioma trials. Neuro Oncol 2017;19(1):12–21.
9. De Groot M, Reijneveld JC, Aronica E, et al. Epilepsy in patients with a brain tumour: focal epilepsy requires focused treatment. Brain 2012;135(Pt 4):1002–16.
10. Duffau H. Diffuse low-grade gliomas and neuroplasticity. Diagn Interv Imaging 2014;95(10):945–55.
11. Tucha O, Smely C, Preier M, et al. Cognitive deficits before treatment among patients with brain tumors. Neurosurgery 2000;47(2):324–33 [discussion: 333–4].
12. Fisher Robert S, Cross JH, French Jacqueline A, et al. Operational classification of seizure types by the International League Against Epilepsy: position paper of the ILAE commission for classification and terminology. Epilepsia 2017;58(4):522–30.
13. Isnard J, Guénot M, Sindou M, et al. Clinical manifestations of insular lobe seizures: a stereo-electroencephalographic study. Epilepsia 2004; 45(9):1079–90.
14. Wu AS, Witgert ME, Lang Frederick F, et al. Neurocognitive function before and after surgery for insular gliomas. J Neurosurg 2011;115(6): 1115–25.
15. Antonsson M, Longoni F, Jakola A, et al. Pre-operative language ability in patients with presumed low-grade glioma. J Neurooncol 2018;137(1):93–102.
16. Duffau H. Cognitive assessment in glioma patients. J Neurosurg 2013;119(5):1348–9.
17. Taphoorn MJ, Klein M. Cognitive deficits in adult patients with brain tumours. Lancet Neurol 2004;3(3): 159–68.
18. Boele FW, Douw L, Reijneveld JC, et al. Health-related quality of life in stable, long-term survivors of low-grade glioma. J Clin Oncol 2015;33(9): 1023–9.
19. Rofes A, Mandonnet E, Godden J, et al. Survey on current cognitive practices within the European Low-Grade Glioma Network: towards a European assessment protocol. Acta Neurochir (Wien) 2017; 159(7):1167–78.
20. Kaloshi G, Psimaras D, Mokhtari K, et al. Supratentorial low-grade gliomas in older patients. Neurology 2009;73(24):2093–8.
21. Mainio A, Hakko H, Niemelä A, et al. The effect of brain tumour laterality on anxiety levels among neurosurgical patients. J Neurol Neurosurg Psychiatr 2003;74(9):1278–82.
22. Drewes C, Sagberg LM, Jakola AS, et al. Quality of life in patients with intracranial tumors: does tumor laterality matter? J Neurosurg 2016;125(6): 1400–7.

23. Struik K, Klein M, Heimans JJ, et al. Fatigue in low-grade glioma. J Neurooncol 2009;92(1):73–8.

24. Potts MB, Smith JS, Molinaro AM, et al. Natural history and surgical management of incidentally discovered low-grade gliomas. J Neurosurg 2012; 116(2):365–72.

25. Pallud J, Mandonnet E. Incidental low-grade gliomas. J Neurosurg 2013;118(3):702–4.

26. Zhang Z-YY, Chan AK, Ng H-KK, et al. Surgically treated incidentally discovered low-grade gliomas are mostly IDH mutated and 1p19q co-deleted with favorable prognosis. Int J Clin Exp Pathol 2014;7(12):8627–36.

27. Cochereau J, Herbet G, Duffau H. Patients with incidental WHO grade II glioma frequently suffer from neuropsychological disturbances. Acta Neurochir (Wien) 2016;158(2):305–12.

28. Smits A, Zetterling M, Lundin M, et al. Neurological impairment linked with cortico-subcortical infiltration of diffuse low-grade gliomas at initial diagnosis supports early brain plasticity. Front Neurol 2015;6:137.

29. Lannin DR, Wang S. Are small breast cancers good because they are small or small because they are good? N Engl J Med 2017;376(23):2286–91.

30. Cochereau J, Herbet G, Rigau V, et al. Acute progression of untreated incidental WHO Grade II glioma to glioblastoma in an asymptomatic patient. J Neurosurg 2016;124(1):141–5.

31. Solheim O, Torsteinsen M, Johannesen TB, et al. Effects of cerebral magnetic resonance imaging in outpatients on observed incidence of intracranial tumors and patient survival: a national observational study. J Neurosurg 2014;120(4): 827–32.

32. Lima GL, Zanello M, Mandonnet E, et al. Incidental diffuse low-grade gliomas: from early detection to preventive neuro-oncological surgery. Neurosurg Rev 2016;39(3):377–84.

33. Pallud J, Mandonnet E, Duffau H, et al. Prognostic value of initial magnetic resonance imaging growth rates for World Health Organization grade II gliomas. Ann Neurol 2006;60(3):380–3.

34. Ricard D, Kaloshi G, Amiel-Benouaich A, et al. Dynamic history of low-grade gliomas before and after temozolomide treatment. Ann Neurol 2007;61(5): 484–90.

35. Van den Bent M, Afra D, de Witte O, et al. Long-term efficacy of early versus delayed radiotherapy for low-grade astrocytoma and oligodendroglioma in adults: the EORTC 22845 randomised trial. Lancet 2005;366(9490):985–90.

36. Baumert BG, Hegi ME, van den Bent MJ, et al. Temozolomide chemotherapy versus radiotherapy in high-risk low-grade glioma (EORTC 22033-26033): a randomised, open-label, phase 3 intergroup study. Lancet Oncol 2016;17(11):1521–32.

37. Reijneveld JC, Taphoorn MJ, Coens C, et al. Health-related quality of life in patients with high-risk low-grade glioma (EORTC 22033-26033): a randomised, open-label, phase 3 intergroup study. Lancet Oncol 2016;17(11):1533–42.

38. Jakola AS, Myrmel KS, Kloster R, et al. Comparison of a strategy favoring early surgical resection vs a strategy favoring watchful waiting in low-grade gliomas. JAMA 2012;308(18):1881–8.

39. Al-Tamimi YZ, Palin MS, Patankar T, et al. Low-grade glioma with foci of early transformation does not necessarily require adjuvant therapy after radical surgical resection. World Neurosurg 2018;110: e346–54.

40. Shaw EG, Wang M, Coons SW, et al. Randomized trial of radiation therapy plus procarbazine, lomustine, and vincristine chemotherapy for supratentorial adult low-grade glioma: initial results of RTOG 9802. J Clin Oncol 2012;30(25): 3065–70.

41. Van den Bent MJ. Chemotherapy for low-grade glioma: when, for whom, which regimen? Curr Opin Neurol 2015;28(6):633–938.

42. Van Thuijl HF, Mazor T, Johnson BE, et al. Evolution of DNA repair defects during malignant progression of low-grade gliomas after temozolomide treatment. Acta Neuropathol 2015;129(4):597–607.

43. Olar A, Sulman EP. Molecular markers in low-grade glioma—toward tumor reclassification. Semin Radiat Oncol 2015;25(3):155–63.

44. Soffietti R, Baumert BG, Bello L, et al. Guidelines on management of low-grade gliomas: report of an EFNS-EANO Task Force. Eur J Neurol 2010;17(9): 1124–33.

45. Miller JJ, Wen PY. Emerging targeted therapies for glioma. Expert Opin Emerg Drugs 2016;21(4): 441–52.

46. Johnson BE, Mazor T, Hong C, et al. Mutational analysis reveals the origin and therapy-driven evolution of recurrent glioma. Science 2014;343(6167): 189–93.

47. Chang EF, Smith JS, Chang SM, et al. Preoperative prognostic classification system for hemispheric low-grade gliomas in adults. J Neurosurg 2008; 109(5):817–24.

48. Pignatti F, van den Bent M, Curran D, et al. Prognostic factors for survival in adult patients with cerebral low-grade glioma. J Clin Oncol 2002;20(8): 2076–84.

49. Gorlia T, Wu W, Wang M, et al. New validated prognostic models and prognostic calculators in patients with low-grade gliomas diagnosed by central pathology review: a pooled analysis of EORTC/RTOG/NCCTG phase III clinical trials. Neuro Oncol 2013; 15(11):1568–79.

50. Daniels TB, Brown PD, Felten SJ, et al. Validation of EORTC prognostic factors for adults with low-grade

glioma: a report using intergroup 86-72-51. Int J Radiat Oncol Biol Phys 2011;81(1):218–24.

51. Pallud J, Audureau E, Blonski M, et al. Epileptic seizures in diffuse low-grade gliomas in adults. Brain 2014;137(Pt 2):449–62.

52. Pallud J, Blonski M, Mandonnet E, et al. Velocity of tumor spontaneous expansion predicts long-term outcomes for diffuse low-grade gliomas. Neuro Oncol 2013;15(5):595–606.

53. Pallud J, Capelle L, Tallandier L, et al. Prognostic significance of imaging contrast enhancement for WHO grade II gliomas. Neuro Oncol 2009;11(2):176–82.

54. Capelle L, Fontaine D, Mandonnet E, et al. Spontaneous and therapeutic prognostic factors in adult hemispheric World Health Organization Grade II gliomas: a series of 1097 cases: clinical article. J Neurosurg 2013;118(6):1157–68.

55. Tang C, Zhang Z-YY, Chen L-CC, et al. Subgroup characteristics of insular low-grade glioma based on clinical and molecular analysis of 42 cases. J Neurooncol 2016;126(3):499–507.

56. Darlix A, Deverdun J, Menjot de Champfleur N, et al. IDH mutation and 1p19q codeletion distinguish two radiological patterns of diffuse low-grade gliomas. J Neurooncol 2017;133(1):37–45.

Diffuse Low-Grade Glioma-Related Epilepsy

Johan Pallud, MD, PhD[a,b,c,d],*, Guy M. McKhann, MD[e]

KEYWORDS

- Diffuse low-grade glioma • Epileptic seizure • Glutamate • GABA • Isocitrate dehydrogenase
- Mammalian target of rapamycin (mTOR) • Surgery • Maximal functional-based resection

KEY POINTS

- Epileptic seizures occur in more than 90% of diffuse low-grade gliomas.
- Epileptic seizures and drug resistance progress during the course of diffuse low-grade gliomas.
- In diffuse low-grade gliomas, multiple epileptogenic foci are located within the peritumoral neocortex infiltrated by isolated glioma cells.
- The glioma-related epileptogenic mechanisms are multifactorial and intermixed and share common mechanisms with glioma growth processes and mechanisms of epileptogenesis in other brain pathologic conditions.
- The main predictors of postoperative seizure control in diffuse low-grade gliomas are a short seizure duration before surgery and a large extent of glioma resection.
- A supratotal resection of a diffuse low-grade glioma (removing the peripheral infiltrated neocortex surrounding the glioma core) can improve postoperative seizure control.
- The presence of epileptic seizures at diagnosis positively affects diffuse low-grade glioma malignant progression-free survival and overall survival.

INTRODUCTION

Epileptic seizures are iconic symptomatic expressions of cerebral gliomas.[1] The origin and mechanisms of human glioma-related epilepsy are multifactorial, intermixed within the same patient, and depend on specific mechanisms related to the tumor itself and to changes within the peritumoral neocortex.[2,3] Epileptic seizure incidence varies with tumor subtype, grade, and location; and one can observe a decrease in epileptogenicity from low-grade gliomas to high-grade gliomas.[1,4] Among the various glioma subtypes, according to the World Health Organization (WHO), diffuse low-grade gliomas (DLGGs) are the most highly epileptogenic[2,3] primary diffuse gliomas in adults. Indeed, epileptic seizures are the most frequent presenting symptoms, and epileptic seizures and drug resistance progress along the natural course of DLGGs.[1] In addition, both epileptic seizures and antiepileptic drug therapy induce cognitive impairments and impair the patient's quality of life, which is a main concern during the long survival of DLGG and may affect the oncological outcomes owing to possible interactions with chemotherapy and possible direct oncological effects.[5–7] Seizure control in DLGG patients is often difficult to achieve by antiepileptic drug therapy alone, and the application of oncological treatments (surgery, radiotherapy, and

Disclosure Statement: J. Pallud has nothing to disclose. G. McKhann receives funding from Citizens United for Research in Epilepsy (CURE).
[a] Department of Neurosurgery, Sainte-Anne Hospital, 1 rue Cabanis, Paris Cedex 14 75674, France; [b] Paris Descartes University, Sorbonne Paris Cité, Paris, France; [c] French Glioma Study Group, Réseau d'Etude des Gliomes, REG, Groland, France; [d] Inserm, U894, Centre Psychiatrie et Neurosciences, Paris, France; [e] Department of Neurological Surgery, Columbia University Medical Center, New York Presbyterian Hospital, New York, NY, USA
* Corresponding author. Service de Neurochirurgie, Hôpital Sainte-Anne, 1 rue Cabanis, Paris Cedex 14 75674, France,
E-mail address: johanpallud@hotmail.com

chemotherapy) significantly helps.[1,8] The identification of predictors of epileptic seizure risk and control in DLGG patients is mandatory to tailor and adapt antiepileptic drugs and oncological treatments on an individual basis.

This article summarizes the incidence and predictors of epilepsy in DLGG in adults; the currently known underlying pathophysiological epileptogenic mechanisms; the impact of oncological treatments, particularly of surgical resection, on epileptic seizures; the predictors of postoperative seizure control; and the impact of epileptic seizures on DLGG outcomes.

EPILEPSY AT DIFFUSE LOW-GRADE GLIOMA DIAGNOSIS
Definition

According to the International League Against Epilepsy, a tumor-related epilepsy is defined as a history of at least 1 epileptic seizure due to the presence of an enduring alteration in the brain (eg, DLGG).[4] No clinical sign of an epileptic seizure is a specific feature of DLGG, and a subtle focal seizure may be missed in patients with cognitive disorders. However, patients with a DLGG typically present with localization-related seizures, depending on the glioma location.[5] Accordingly, patients present mainly with focal seizures (45%–95%).[1,9]

Incidence and Risk Factors of Epilepsy at Diagnosis

Epileptic seizure is the most frequent presenting sign of DLGG, occurring in more than 80% of cases, and the most frequent sign at diagnosis, occurring in more than 90% of cases.[1,2,6,7] The observation of cohorts of subjects with an incidentally discovered DLGG highlights that epileptic seizures occur during the patient follow-up concomitantly to the glioma growth, in the absence of oncological treatment.[10,11] A series of 208 subjects in whom no oncological treatment was administered after DLGG diagnosis highlights an increase of drug-resistant seizures along the natural course of the DLGG.[1] This illustrates that epileptic seizures progress during the natural course of DLGG.

Seizure history and control rates vary among DLGG patients, depending on the presence of risk factors. Regarding patient-related risk factors, the risk of seizures decreases with increased patient age and is increased in male patients.[1,8] Regarding glioma-related risk factors, tumor location influences the risk for epilepsy. The seizure risk increases in DLGGs invading the neocortex and decreases in deeply located tumors.[12] DLGGs involving the frontal, temporal, insular, and parietal lobes are more commonly associated with seizures

than occipital DLGGs. DLGG proximity to eloquent cortex also increases seizure frequency.[1] This can be explained by the variation of DLGG subtypes and the intrinsic epileptogenicity of particular cerebral lobes.[1,13] As an example, paralimbic DLGG locations, particularly insular DLGGs, and frontocentral DLGGs are associated with an increased seizure risk.[1,14–20] The risk of seizure increases with the tumor volume in DLGGs, possibly due to the slow growth of the DLGG that allows epileptogenic mechanisms to develop concomitantly with neuroplasticity, in contrast to gliomas of a higher grade of malignancy.[1,9]

The influence of histopathological subtypes and biomolecular markers on the risk of seizures is difficult to assess because the definition of DLGG has varied with the different versions of the WHO classifications over time. With the knowledge of this limitation, epileptic seizures seem more common in oligodendrogliomas and in mixed gliomas than in astrocytomas in the University of California, San Francisco (UCSF) experience[10] and in the Glioma International Case Control Study[11]; whereas in 3 large series from different institutions, the histopathological subtype did not significantly affect the seizure risk.[1,21,22] The presence of an isocitrate dehydrogenase (IDH)1 or IDH2 mutation seems associated with a higher risk of seizures in DLGG.[23–26] Two recent meta-analyses, 1 including 772 and 1 including 540 DLGG subjects (72% and 78% with an IDH1 mutation, respectively) identified IDH1 mutation to be correlated with a higher risk of preoperative epileptic seizures.[14,27] Another recent systematic review and meta-analysis including 1585 subjects (44% with an IDH1 or IDH2 mutation) identified IDH1 or IDH2 mutation to be correlated with a higher risk of epileptic seizures preoperatively in DLGG only but not in high-grade gliomas, with similar findings for IDH1 mutations as for IDH2 mutations.[15] No significant association between the presence of the 1p19q codeletion and seizure risk has been observed in DLGG[1,16,17] in contrast to the higher seizure frequency that has been observed in oligodendrogliomas. The absence of a 19q deletion is associated with a higher risk of seizures in DLGG in 1 study.[17] Two large studies focused on DLGG found no correlation between seizure risk and biomolecular markers.[1,21]

Incidence and Risk Factors of Uncontrolled Epilepsy at Diagnosis

The International League Against Epilepsy commission on therapeutic strategies defines uncontrolled seizures or refractory epilepsy as an epilepsy that is not controlled by 2 tolerated and appropriately chosen and used antiepileptic drugs schedules, whether as monotherapies or in combination.[18] The predictors of uncontrolled seizures are difficult to assess between studies because the definition of seizure control varies between Engel class 1A, a much more stringent outcome grading that requires patients to be completely seizure-free, and Engel class 1, which includes patients with simple partial postoperative seizures and postoperative drug withdrawal seizures.[19]

In general, for patients with DLGGs, the rates of uncontrolled seizures before oncological treatment vary from 15% to 50%.[1,10,21] This can be attributed to the varying time interval between a patient's first seizure and oncological treatment because epileptic seizures and drug resistance frequently increase from the time seizures begin to the time of DLGG diagnosis, and continue to increase over time as the DLGG grows.[1] Indeed, in a cohort of 208 subjects with a histologically proven and untreated DLGG, uncontrolled epileptic seizures progressed despite antiepileptic drugs. The rates of uncontrolled epileptic seizures despite antiepileptic drugs increased from 13% at the time of histopathological diagnosis to 40% at a mean of 34 months of follow-up without oncological treatment.[1] In addition, uncontrolled seizures progressed during the course of treated DLGG, despite antiepileptic drug therapy and oncological treatments: 2% at imaging discovery, 15% at histopathological diagnosis, 33% after first-line oncological treatment, and more than 40% at malignant transformation.[1] In 1 study, subjects with a astrocytoma DLGG subtype presented with more uncontrolled epileptic seizures.[11]

Glioma-Related Epileptogenicity

When studying the mechanisms of human glioma-related epilepsy in diffuse gliomas as a whole, whatever the grade of malignancy, mounting evidence suggests that glioma growth stimulates seizures and that seizures encourage glioma growth, leading to the concept that glioma growth and epileptic seizures share common underlying mechanisms.[20] Epileptogenic mechanisms seem multifactorial and intermixed between mechanisms related to the tumor itself and mechanisms related to modifications of the tumor microenvironment.[1–3,28] Several mechanisms may be present within the same glioma patient and mechanisms seem to vary between DLGG patients and high-grade gliomas patients.

Cortical Foci of Glioma-Related Epilepsy

Preoperative electrophysiological investigations (magnetoencephalography, surface electroence

phalography [EEG], stereo-EEG) and intraoperative electrophysiological investigations (direct electrocorticography [ECoG], transcorticography) record epileptic activities mainly within the peritumoral neocortex.[2,29] Ex vivo electrophysiological explorations of spatially oriented human samples have shown that these activities arise mainly within the supragranular cortical layers of the peritumoral neocortex infiltrated by glioma cells but not in the glioma core.[30] As for other diffuse gliomas, the DLGG foci of epileptic activity are located at the frontier between the glioma per se and the surrounding functional neocortex. This peritumoral neocortex microscopically invaded by isolated glioma cells is the anatomic key structure for DLGG-related epileptogenesis.

Epileptogenic Mechanisms Related to Glioma Properties

Because a DLGG is a space-occupying mass, mechanical effects may contribute to produce epileptic activities.[3] Mass effect and edema may induce microcirculation impairments and cerebral hypoperfusion, which are responsible for focal ischemic changes.[31] The DLGG's slow growth and infiltration may isolate and cause deafferentation of the corticosubcortical local and distant networks, leading to epileptogenicity.[32,33] Rarely in DLGG, an acute tissue event, including hemorrhage or necrosis, may participate in epileptogenesis.[33] However, the DLGG literature generally lacks significant correlations between seizures and tumor volume, mass effect, edema, necrosis, or histopathological and biomolecular findings. Instead, multiple studies demonstrate positive correlations between seizures and cortex involvement and tumor location. Taken together, these cumulative results suggest that DLGG epileptogenicity is mainly triggered by interactions between the tumor and the neocortex rather than by intrinsic tumor properties alone.[1,3,31,32]

Structural reorganization and functional deafferentation within the peritumoral neocortex (neuronal loss, glial loss, neurogenesis, reactive astrogliosis, neuronal plasticity) have been described.[31–33] Accordingly, magnetoencephalography has shown that gliomas disrupt functional connectivity of brain networks within peritumoral and distant brain areas.[32] Such changes may induce alterations in local neuronal networks, resulting in a reduction of inhibitory pathways and an increase of excitatory ones. Ultimately this imbalance between excitation and inhibition eventually results in epileptogenicity.

Glioma cells predate their surrounding environment by recruiting nonglioma cells (astrocytes, microglia, stromal cells) that provide resources and growth advantage to facilitate tumor progression. Glioma cells activate and attract neighboring microglia that, in turn, can modulate glioma biology: activated microglia enhance glioma cells' migration abilities. The pathologic disruption of the blood brain barrier that exposes the brain to blood serum components, such as glutamate, fibrinogen, and albumin, together with the release of vascular endothelial growth factor,[23] is classically not observed in DLGG.

Epileptogenic Mechanisms Related to Peritumoral Changes

Glutamate homeostasis is impaired in the vicinity of diffuse gliomas. Glioma cells lack sodium (Na^+)-dependent excitatory amino acid transporters 1 and 2, leading to a decrease in glutamate uptake,[24,32] and express the system Xc-cystine glutamate transporter, leading to an increase in glutamate release.[34–38] This results in highly elevated and sustained extracellular glutamate concentrations (>100 μm) that are up to 10-fold higher than normal. In addition, nontumoral astrocytes and activated microglia of the peritumoral neocortex display impaired glutamate clearance abilities with reduced extracellular glutamate uptake and increased glutamate release.[23] In parallel, mutations of the IDH genes that are predominant in DLGG lead to conversion of isocitrate to D-2-hydroxyglutarate rather than to α-ketoglutarate.[25] Consequently, D-2-hydroxyglutarate accumulates in glioma cells and the extracellular space, where it is thought to act as a glutamate receptor agonist owing to its steric analogy to glutamate.[20,26] This possibly explains why IDH mutations in DLGG are associated with a higher risk of epileptic seizures in clinical practice.[1,24,26,39]

DLGG epileptogenicity is likely at least partially related to excessive local glutamatergic excitatory neurotransmission. The excessive extracellular glutamate in the glioma microenvironment may induce seizures through the facilitation of pathologic pyramidal cells synchronization.[40] Experimentation on glioma-bearing mice confirmed that peritumoral neuronal hyperexcitability was attributable to glutamate release by glioma cells via the system Xc-cystine glutamate transporter.[39] In human glioma subjects, a recent study identified that a high system Xc-cystine glutamate transporter expression is associated with seizures at the time of diagnosis but not with uncontrolled seizures.[41] Interestingly, the system Xc-cystine glutamate transporter seems to be more expressed in IDH-wildtype high-grade gliomas than in IDH-

mutated DLGG,[41] suggesting that the glutamatergic-mediated epileptogenicity has a different origin in high-grade gliomas (glutamate release from glioma cells with the system Xc-cystine glutamate transporter) than in DLGG (D-2-hydroxyglutarate accumulation in the extracellular space acting as a glutamate receptor agonist).

Gamma-aminobutyric (GABA)-ergic signaling is also impaired in the vicinity of diffuse gliomas. The peritumoral neocortex presents reduced GABAergic inhibitory anatomic pathways with a loss of GABAergic interneurons[42] and a reduction of inhibitory synapses onto pyramidal cells.[43] These alterations result in a weakening of GABAergic inhibitory function within peritumoral neocortex.[23,28,32,39] In addition, dysregulation of intracellular chloride (Cl^-) in peritumoral neocortex influences neuronal responses to GABA. In healthy mature neurons, intracellular Cl^- is maintained at low levels by activation of the potassium (K^+)-Cl^- cotransporter 2 (KCC2), which extrudes Cl^- with K^+ out of neurons, and repression of the Na^+-K^+-Cl^- cotransporter 1 (NKCC1), which uptakes Cl^-, Na^+, and K^+ into neurons.[20] In healthy mature neurons, activation of GABA receptors causes Cl^- influx that hyperpolarizes cells and inhibits neuronal activity. In contrast, in gliomas, an aberrant downregulation of KCC2 and upregulation of NKCC1 leads to accumulation of intracellular Cl^-, which contributes to both glioma proliferation and migration and to epileptic activity.[20,29,30] The intracellular Cl^- accumulation of glioma cells, up to approximately 100 mM, 10-fold higher than normal, is actively maintained by the NKCC1,[44] which is highly expressed in glioma cells.[30,45,46] About 60% of neurons (pyramidal cells) within peritumoral cortex are affected by such Cl^- homeostasis dysregulation.[30,47] This disruption is caused by upregulated expression of NKCC1 and downregulated expression of KCC2 in these neurons.[44,48–51] GABA activation of these peritumoral pyramidal neurons with elevated intracellular Cl^- induces excitatory depolarization rather than the inhibitory neuronal hyperpolarization that is normally seen in the adult brain in response to $GABA_A$ activation, promoting epileptogenesis.[30]

Epileptogenicity in peritumoral tissue likely results from both pathologic glutamate release and GABA-mediated disinhibition of surrounding pyramidal cells. Interestingly, many features of peritumoral epileptiform activity are similar to those seen in nontumoral genetic and acquired human epilepsies, suggesting a convergence of pathologic mechanisms. Drugs that target cellular membrane K^+-Cl^- cotransporters and delivery mechanisms aimed at delivering these drugs specifically to peritumoral tissue represent possible clinical and technological patient treatment advances that could both improve seizure control and promote survival in glioma patients.

There are several other potential mechanisms of human brain epileptogenicity shared between glioma tissue and other brain pathologic conditions, such as mesial temporal sclerosis and tuberous sclerosis complex. K^+ buffering is impaired in both gliomas and sclerotic mesial temporal tissue. In gliomas, there is a loss of expression of Kir4.1 channels in the plasma membrane of cells, a channel that is required for cell proliferation in glioma cells and for K^+ uptake in normal astrocytes.[52] The resulting high extracellular K^+ concentration together with other local perturbations, such as the alkalization of the peritumoral neocortex[31] and the alterations in the function of peritumoral glial cell gap junction function,[31,32] may increase the excitability of surrounding pyramidal cells and favor epileptogenesis.

Activation of the mammalian target of rapamycin (mTOR) pathway has been implicated in both gliomagenesis and tumor progression,[34–36] as well as in epileptogenesis of various causes.[37,38,53,54] mTOR activity is increased in peritumoral neurons in human glioma specimens compared with neurons in control neocortex and may contribute to glioma epileptogenesis.[55] Interestingly, neuronal activity has been shown to induce glioma progenitor cell proliferation, also via activation of the mTOR pathway.[56] Thus, tumor growth into peritumoral brain likely results in glioma epileptogenesis, whereas neuronal activity in a peritumoral brain may in turn promote tumor proliferation, resulting in a vicious cycle of tumor progression and morbidity. The mTOR pathway represents a targetable checkpoint in glioma proliferation, epileptogenesis, and pathogenesis. This pathway is currently being studied to determine whether preoperative administration of a mTOR inhibitor to glioma patients can decrease peritumoral neuronal mTOR expression and lessen the abnormal hyperexcitability that is found in peritumoral brain. mTOR inhibitors are already commonly used clinically in many settings, with a good safety profile.

Impact of Oncological Treatments on Seizure Control

Oncological treatments (surgery, radiotherapy, chemotherapy) affect seizure control of DLGG-related epilepsy.

Surgical resection

The impact of surgical resection on DLGG-related seizures is illustrated in **Fig. 1**. Surgical resection provides seizure control in 36% to 100% of diffuse DLGGs.[57–59] Literature reviews[60,61] identified the extent of resection as the main predictor of postoperative seizure control. These results were reproduced in the largest study dedicated to epileptic seizures in supratentorial DLGG in adults from the French Glioma Network (1509 cases) in which age and the extent of resection were independent predictors of postoperative seizure control; whereas history of seizures at diagnosis, and parietal and insular locations, were independent predictors of postoperative uncontrolled seizures.[1] The Glioma International Case Control Study identified that gross total resection is associated with reduced seizure frequency postoperatively.[11] Other predictors of postoperative uncontrolled seizures are the presence of a preoperative neurologic deficit, the DLGG location,[1,6,22,30,61–63] and a younger age at surgery together with a shorter seizure duration before surgery.[1,21,22,30,61,64,65] Of interest, 1 study points to a tumor's IDH mutational status as associated with more severe uncontrolled seizures postoperatively.[66] The concentration of glutamate in the DLGG microenvironment has been shown not to be associated with postoperative seizures.[48]

The extent of resection is a primary predictor of postoperative seizure control in DLGG patients. The probability of seizure control increases with the extent of resection: uncontrolled seizures in 44% following biopsy, in 40% following partial resection, in 32% following subtotal resection, and in 16% following total resection.[1] The recent experience of the Barrow Neurologic Institute clarified the extent of resection threshold for postoperative seizure control.[59] In a series of 128 newly-diagnosed DLGGs, they reported that the proportion of postoperative seizure control increased in proportion to the extent of resection, and that seizure control can be attained when an extent of resection higher than 80% is achieved.[59] Intraoperative functional mapping using direct electrical cortical and subcortical stimulation under awake conditions does not increase the risk of early and late postoperative seizures.[67–69] When observed, the occurrence of intraoperative seizures does not necessitate aborting glioma surgery in most instances.[49,50,70]

A major issue related to glioma surgery is that independent epileptogenic foci can be nested within extratumoral cortical areas that are grossly free of tumor. This may explain why some patients still suffer from uncontrolled seizures postoperatively, even after a total DLGG resection, based on postoperative MRI. In this setting, the removal of the putative epileptogenic foci beyond the tumor, including the hippocampal formation for paralimbic DLGGs, could lead to improved seizure

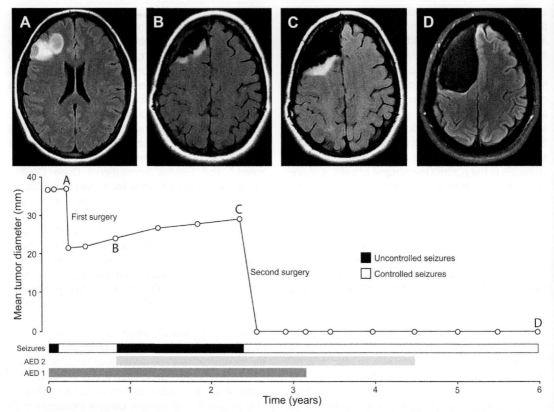

Fig. 1. The impact of surgical resection on DLGG-related epileptic seizure. A 33-year-old right-handed woman presented with partial motor and secondary generalized epileptic seizures controlled with 1 antiepileptic drug (AED) and a right frontal nonenhanced mass with spontaneous growth on MRI (Panel A). A subtotal resection was performed under general anesthesia and confirmed the diagnosis of a WHO grade II IDH1 mutated oligodendroglioma (Panel B). Five months after surgery, epileptic seizures recurred, requiring the introduction of AED 2 and the residual tumor grew on MRI (Panel C). Epileptic seizures remained uncontrolled despite 2 AEDs. Following a dedicated preoperative cognitive rehabilitation, a second surgical resection was performed using intraoperative functional mapping with direct cortical and subcortical electrostimulations under awake condition and allowed a supratotal resection beyond MRI-defined abnormalities. Following this second surgery, epileptic seizures were controlled, AED 1 was stopped at 6 postoperative months and AED 2 was stopped at 30 postoperative months. At 6 years postoperative follow-up, the patient was seizure-free, no glioma recurrence was observed (Panel D), and cognitive evaluation demonstrated an improvement compared with preoperative evaluation.

outcomes.[51,58] Similarly, the emerging concept of supratotal resection (ie, removing a margin beyond MRI-defined abnormalities until functional cortico-subcortical boundaries are reached)[71] for better seizure control has been proposed.[60,61] It relies on the possible removal of the putative epileptogenic foci through a supratotal resection beyond MRI-defined abnormalities.[30] Second surgery using intraoperative functional mapping can be useful for seizure control of DLGG in cases with an initial partial removal[12,62,72] or at tumor progression.[63] A series from the Duffau group previously demonstrated that reoperation using intraoperative functional cortical and subcortical mapping of DLGG located within eloquent areas provided both better DLGG control and better seizure control.[72] Preoperative neoadjuvant chemotherapy

can be considered before DLGG surgical removal; preliminary studies are encouraging.[64,65] Finally, the use of intraoperative ECoG monitoring during DLGG surgery to identify epileptogenic foci may further improve postoperative seizure control.[73,74] However, previous series led to varying results. It is acknowledged that the cases in which ECoG was used were associated with more severe and refractory epilepsy.[58] Taken together, these data suggest that the extent of resection is a main prognostic parameter of DLGG postoperative seizure control that must be achieved for both epileptological and oncological purposes.

Radiotherapy
The impact of radiotherapy on DLGG-related seizures is illustrated in **Fig. 2**. The impact of

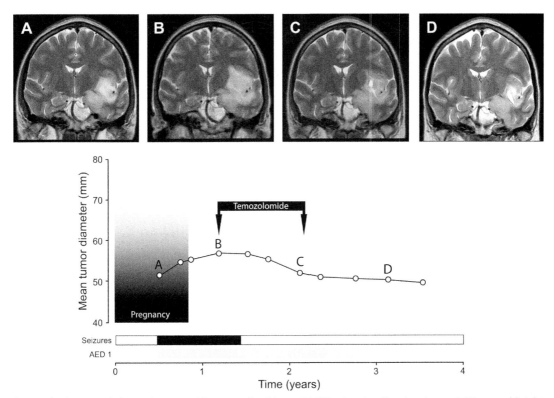

Fig. 2. The impact of chemotherapy with temozolomide on DLGG-related epileptic seizure. A 37-year-old right-handed woman presented with generalized tonicoclonic seizures at 5 months of pregnancy (Panel A). Seizures remained uncontrolled despite 1 AED and the end of pregnancy was uneventful. A stereotactic biopsy was performed 3 months after delivery and confirmed the diagnosis of a WHO grade II IDH mutated astrocytoma (Panel B). Chemotherapy with temozolomide was started 7 months after delivery (12 cycles for 1 year), allowing epileptic seizure control after 3 cycles (Panel C). The AED was arrested 7 months after the end of chemotherapy. At 3.5 years postoperative follow-up, the patient was seizure-free and no glioma recurrence was observed (Panel D).

radiotherapy on DLGG-related seizures is supported by limited data.[6,75] Conventional radiotherapy has been reported to improve seizure control in about 75% of DLGG patients with uncontrolled seizures.[6] A retrospective series of 33 DLGGs demonstrated a reduction of 50% or more of the seizure frequency in 75% of cases following radiotherapy; 35% of subjects had controlled seizures at 1 year postradiotherapy.[75] Of note, seizure reduction usually begins early following radiotherapy and precedes the tumor shrinkage on MRI.[75,76] The time to radiotherapy seems to affect the resultant seizure control. The European Organisation for Research and Treatment of Cancer 22845 phase III trial, which compared early radiotherapy versus observation and radiotherapy at progression in DLGG, demonstrated that 25% of subjects who were irradiated early had uncontrolled seizures, compared with 41% of subjects who were not irradiated early.[67] This finding is consistent with the observation discussed previously of seizure progression along the DLGG clinical course in the absence of oncological treatment. Of note, no difference in seizure control has been observed between high (59.4 Gy) and low (45 Gy) doses of radiotherapy.[68,69]

Chemotherapy

The impact of chemotherapy on DLGG-related seizures is illustrated in **Fig. 3**. The impact of chemotherapy with alkylating agents on DLGG-related seizures is documented. Temozolomide allows a reduction of the seizure frequency in 50% to 60% of subjects, 20% to 40% of them being seizure-free.[6,77–79] A series of 39 DLGG subjects demonstrated a reduction of the seizure frequency of 50% or more in 60% of subjects following temozolomide compared with 13% in subjects with antiepileptic drug therapy only.[80] A series on insular DLGGs demonstrated a reduction of seizure frequency in 100% of subjects following temozolomide, with 14% of them being seizure-free compared with seizure reduction of 30% in subjects with antiepileptic drug therapy only.[62] A preoperative neoadjuvant chemotherapy with

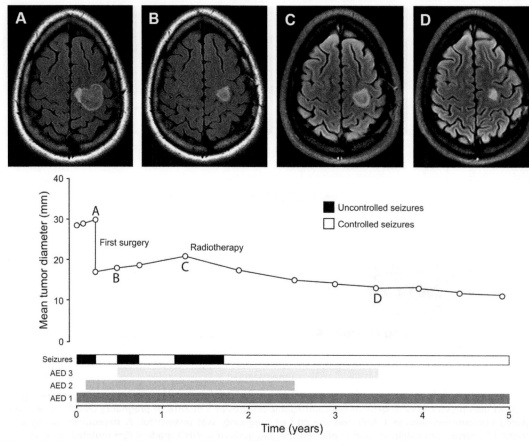

Fig. 3. The impact of radiotherapy on DLGG-related epileptic seizure. A 26-year-old right-handed woman presented with simple partial motor epileptic seizures that remained uncontrolled despite 2 AEDs and a left frontal nonenhanced mass with spontaneous growth on MRI (Panel A). A partial resection was performed using intraoperative functional mapping with direct cortical and subcortical electrostimulations under awake condition and confirmed the diagnosis of a WHO grade II IDH mutated mixed glioma (Panel B). Five months after surgery, epileptic seizures recurred, requiring the introduction of AED 3 and the residual tumor grew on MRI. At 1 postoperative year, epileptic seizures recurred and remained uncontrolled despite 3 AEDs (Panel C). A conformational external radiotherapy was performed (50.4 Gy), allowing epileptic seizure control 9 months after radiotherapy and AED 2 arrest about 1 year after radiotherapy and AED 3 arrest about 2 years after radiotherapy. At 5 years postoperative follow-up, the patient was seizure-free and no glioma recurrence was observed (Panel D).

temozolomide demonstrated a reduction of the seizure frequency in 90% of cases, 50% of them being seizure-free.[64,65] Interestingly, following surgery and neoadjuvant temozolomide, a reduction of the seizure frequency was observed in 100% of cases, 70% of them being seizure-free.[64] To date, no significant correlation between seizure response and 1p/19q codeletion status and DLGG subtype has been reported.[6] Similar to radiotherapy, the temozolomide-induced reduction of seizure frequency precedes the tumor response seen on imaging follow-up and seems correlated with survival in DLGG patients.[81]

Chemotherapy with procarbazine plus Chlorethyl-Cyclohexyl-Nitroso-Urea (CCNU) plus vincristine (PCV) allows a reduction of seizure frequency in up to 100% of patients, with up to 60% of them becoming seizure-free.[82] A series of 33 DLGG demonstrated a reduction of seizure frequency in 53% and total seizure control in 31% of subjects following PCV chemotherapy.[83] Alkylating agents seem promising as therapeutic adjuncts to improve seizure control, in addition to their oncological impact, in DLGG patients.

Prognostic Significance of Epileptic Seizures

Epileptic seizures and glioma progression
Clinical practice has taught that recurrent seizures following an initial seizure-free period, the occurrence of new seizures, or an increase in seizure frequency in a patient with a treated DLGG can be the first sign of tumor progression and warrants imaging investigation.[5,12] At glioma

progression, seizures often recur before the detection of an actual progression on imaging follow-up[84] and 1 study reports a 3-month interval between seizure recurrence and imaging diagnosis of glioma progression.[63] In cases in which an EEG follow-up was available, glioma-related electrophysiological alterations were observed in nearly all progressive gliomas. The quantified glioma growth on MRI in pregnant patients harboring a DLGG showed a significant increase in growth rate compared with corresponding pre-pregnancy measures. Also, 40% of the subjects reported a simultaneous increase in seizure frequency, again illustrating the link glioma growth and seizures during the follow-up of treated DLGG patients.[73,74] As a practical consequence, the accurate and reproducible evaluation of seizure control during the postoperative follow-up of DLGG is important because it can serve as a surrogate adjunctive metric of tumor response in DLGG patients.[81,85]

Epileptic seizures and survivals

In DLGG patients, the presence of seizures at diagnosis is associated with more favorable outcomes.[1,12] In the largest study dedicated to epileptic seizures in supratentorial DLGG in adults from the French Glioma Network (1509 cases), a history of epileptic seizure at diagnosis was an independent predictor for overall survival. The overall survivals were about 90 months and 50 months in DLGG patients with and without a history of epileptic seizure at diagnosis, respectively.[1] The prognostic significance of epileptic seizures in malignant transformation is less documented; however, in the same study, a history of epileptic seizure at diagnosis was an independent predictor for malignant transformation: the malignant-free survivals were about 65 months and 40 months in DLGG patients with and without a history of epileptic seizure at diagnosis, respectively.[1]

Altogether, the presence of epileptic seizure independently and positively affect DLGG prognosis.

REFERENCES

1. Pallud J, Audureau E, Blonski M, et al. Epileptic seizures in diffuse low-grade gliomas in adults. Brain 2014;137(Pt 2):449–62.
2. van Breemen MSM, Wilms EB, Vecht CJ. Epilepsy in patients with brain tumours: epidemiology, mechanisms, and management. Lancet Neurol 2007;6(5):421–30.
3. Pallud J, Capelle L, Huberfeld G. Tumoral epileptogenicity: how does it happen? Epilepsia 2013;54(Suppl.9):29–33.
4. Fisher RS, van Emde Boas W, Blume W, et al. Epileptic seizures and epilepsy: definitions proposed by the International League Against Epilepsy (ILAE) and the International Bureau for Epilepsy (IBE). Epilepsia 2005;46(4):470–2.
5. Vercueil L. Brain tumor epilepsy: a reappraisal and six remaining issues to be debated. Rev Neurol (Paris) 2011;167(10):751–61.
6. Ruda R, Bello L, Duffau H, et al. Seizures in low-grade gliomas: natural history, pathogenesis, and outcome after treatments. Neuro Oncol 2012;14(suppl 4):iv55–64.
7. Soffietti R, Baumert BG, Bello L, et al. Guidelines on management of low-grade gliomas: report of an EFNS-EANO* task force. Eur J Neurol 2010;17(9):1124–33.
8. Brogna C, Gil Robles S, Duffau H. Brain tumors and epilepsy. Expert Rev Neurother 2008;8(6):941–55.
9. Lee JW, Wen PY, Hurwitz S, et al. Morphological characteristics of brain tumors causing seizures. Arch Neurol 2010;67(3):336–42.
10. Chang EF, Potts MB, Keles GE, et al. Seizure characteristics and control following resection in 332 patients with low-grade gliomas. J Neurosurg 2008;108(2):227–35.
11. Berntsson SG, Merrell RT, Amirian ES, et al. Glioma-related seizures in relation to histopathological subtypes: a report from the glioma international case-control study. J Neurol 2018;265(6):1432–42.
12. Smits A, Duffau H. Seizures and the natural history of WHO grade II gliomas: a review. Neurosurgery 2011;68(5):1326–33.
13. Duffau H, Capelle L. Preferential brain locations of low-grade gliomas. Cancer 2004;100(12):2622–6.
14. Wang Z-F, Chen H-L. Relationship between IDH1 mutation and preoperative seizure in low-grade gliomas: a meta-analysis. Clin Neurol Neurosurg 2016;148:79–84.
15. Phan K, Ng W, Lu VM, et al. Association between IDH1 and IDH2 mutations and preoperative seizures in patients with low-grade versus high-grade glioma: a systematic review and meta-analysis. World Neurosurg 2018;111:e539–45.
16. Mulligan L, Ryan E, O'Brien M, et al. Genetic features of oligodendrogliomas and presence of seizures. The relationship of seizures and genetics in LGOs. Clin Neuropathol 2014;33(4):292–8.
17. Huang L, You G, Jiang T, et al. Correlation between tumor-related seizures and molecular genetic profile in 103 Chinese patients with low-grade gliomas: a preliminary study. J Neurol Sci 2011;302(1–2):63–7.
18. Kwan P, Arzimanoglou A, Berg AT, et al. Definition of drug resistant epilepsy: consensus proposal by the ad hoc task force of the ILAE commission on therapeutic strategies. Epilepsia 2009;51(6):1069–77.
19. Wieser HG, Blume WT, Fish D, et al. ILAE commission report. Proposal for a new classification of

outcome with respect to epileptic seizures following epilepsy surgery. Epilepsia 2001;42:282–6.

20. Huberfeld G, Vecht CJ. Seizures and gliomas — towards a single therapeutic approach. Nat Rev Neurol 2016;12(4):204–16.

21. You G, Sha Z-Y, Yan W, et al. Seizure characteristics and outcomes in 508 Chinese adult patients undergoing primary resection of low-grade gliomas: a clinicopathological study. Neuro Oncol 2012;14(2): 230–41.

22. Yuan Y, Xiang W, Yanhui L, et al. Ki-67 overexpression in WHO grade II gliomas is associated with poor postoperative seizure control. Seizure 2013; 22(10):877–81.

23. Buckingham SC, Robel S. Glutamate and tumor-associated epilepsy: Glial cell dysfunction in the peritumoral environment. Neurochem Int 2013; 63(7):696–701.

24. Savaskan NE, Heckel A, Hahnen E, et al. Small interfering RNA–mediated xCT silencing in gliomas inhibits neurodegeneration and alleviates brain edema. Nat Med 2008;14(6):629–32.

25. Sanson M, Marie Y, Paris S, et al. Isocitrate dehydrogenase 1 codon 132 mutation is an important prognostic biomarker in gliomas. J Clin Oncol 2009; 27(25):4150–4.

26. Andronesi OC, Kim GS, Gerstner E, et al. Detection of 2-hydroxyglutarate in IDH-mutated glioma patients by in vivo spectral-editing and 2D correlation magnetic resonance spectroscopy. Sci Transl Med 2012;4(116):116ra4.

27. Li Y, Shan X, Wu Z, et al. IDH1 mutation is associated with a higher preoperative seizure incidence in low-grade glioma: a systematic review and meta-analysis. Seizure 2018;55:76–82.

28. Bianchi L, De Micheli E, Bricolo A, et al. Extracellular levels of amino acids and choline in human high grade gliomas: an intraoperative microdialysis study. Neurochem Res 2004;29(1):325–34.

29. Habela CW, Ernest NJ, Swindall AF, et al. Chloride accumulation drives volume dynamics underlying cell proliferation and migration. J Neurophysiol 2009;101(2):750–7.

30. Pallud J, Le Van Quyen M, Bielle F, et al. Cortical GABAergic excitation contributes to epileptic activities around human glioma. Sci Transl Med 2014; 6(244):244ra89.

31. Beaumont A, Whittle IR. The pathogenesis of tumour associated epilepsy. Acta Neurochir (Wien) 2000; 142(1):1–15.

32. de Groot M, Reijneveld JC, Aronica E, et al. Epilepsy in patients with a brain tumour: focal epilepsy requires focused treatment. Brain 2012;135(Pt 4):1002–16.

33. Shamji MF, Fric-Shamji EC, Benoit BG. Brain tumors and epilepsy: pathophysiology of peritumoral changes. Neurosurg Rev 2009;32(3):275–84 [discussion: 284–6].

34. Pachow D, Wick W, Gutmann DH, et al. The mTOR signaling pathway as a treatment target for intracranial neoplasms. Neuro Oncol 2015;17(2):189–99.

35. Kwiatkowska A, Symons M. Signaling determinants of glioma cell invasion. Adv Exp Med Biol 2013; 986(Chapter 7):121–41.

36. Masui K, Cloughesy TF, Mischel PS. Review: molecular pathology in adult high-grade gliomas: from molecular diagnostics to target therapies. Neuropathol Appl Neurobiol 2012;38(3):271–91.

37. Lipton JO, Sahin M. The neurology of mTOR. Neuron 2014;84(2):275–91.

38. Wong M. Mammalian target of rapamycin (mTOR) pathways in neurological diseases. Biomed J 2013;36(2):40–50.

39. Buckingham SC, Campbell SL, Haas BR, et al. Glutamate release by primary brain tumors induces epileptic activity. Nat Med 2011;17(10):1269–74.

40. De Groot J, Sontheimer H. Glutamate and the biology of gliomas. Glia 2011;59(8):1181–9.

41. Sørensen MF, Heimisdóttir SB, Sørensen MD, et al. High expression of cystine-glutamate antiporter xCT (SLC7A11) is an independent biomarker for epileptic seizures at diagnosis in glioma. J Neurooncol 2018;138(1):49–53.

42. Haglund MM, Berger MS, Kunkel DD, et al. Changes in gamma-aminobutyric acid and somatostatin in epileptic cortex associated with low-grade gliomas. J Neurosurg 1992;77(2):209–16.

43. Marco P, Sola RG, Ramón Y, et al. Loss of inhibitory synapses on the soma and axon initial segment of pyramidal cells in human epileptic peritumoural neocortex: implications for epilepsy. Brain Res Bull 1997;44(1):47–66.

44. Haas BR, Sontheimer H. Inhibition of the sodium-potassium-chloride cotransporter isoform-1 reduces glioma invasion. Cancer Res 2010;70(13): 5597–606.

45. Conti L, Palma E, Roseti C, et al. Anomalous levels of Cl- transporters cause a decrease of GABAergic inhibition in human peritumoral epileptic cortex. Epilepsia 2011;52(9):1635–44.

46. Garzon-Muvdi T, Schiapparelli P, Ap Rhys C, et al. Regulation of brain tumor dispersal by NKCC1 through a novel role in focal adhesion regulation. PLoS Biol 2012;10(5):e1001320.

47. Campbell SL, Robel S, Cuddapah VA, et al. GABAergic disinhibition and impaired KCC2 cotransporter activity underlie tumor-associated epilepsy. Glia 2014;63(1):23–36.

48. Neal A, Yuen T, Bjorksten AR, et al. Peritumoural glutamate correlates with post-operative seizures in supratentorial gliomas. J Neurooncol 2016; 129(2):259–67.

49. Pallud J, Rigaux-Viode O, Corns R, et al. Direct electrical bipolar electrostimulation for functional cortical and subcortical cerebral mapping in awake

craniotomy. Practical considerations. Neurochirurgie 2017;63(3):164–74.

50. Spena G, Schucht P, Seidel K, et al. Brain tumors in eloquent areas: a European multicenter survey of intraoperative mapping techniques, intraoperative seizures occurrence, and antiepileptic drug prophylaxis. Neurosurg Rev 2017;40(2):287–98.

51. Ghareeb F, Duffau H. Intractable epilepsy in paralimbic Word Health Organization Grade II gliomas: should the hippocampus be resected when not invaded by the tumor? J Neurosurg 2012;116(6): 1226–34.

52. Olsen ML, Sontheimer H. Functional implications for Kir4.1 channels in glial biology: from K+ buffering to cell differentiation. J Neurochem 2008;107(3): 589–601.

53. Sosunov AA, Wu X, McGovern RA, et al. The mTOR pathway is activated in glial cells in mesial temporal sclerosis. Epilepsia 2012;53(Suppl. 9):78–86.

54. Meng X-F, Yu J-T, Song J-H, et al. Role of the mTOR signaling pathway in epilepsy. J Neurol Sci 2013; 332(1–2):4–15.

55. Yuan Y, Xiang W, Yanhui L, et al. Activation of the mTOR signaling pathway in peritumoral tissues can cause glioma-associated seizures. Neurol Sci 2017;38(1):61–6.

56. Venkatesh HS, Johung TB, Caretti V, et al. Neuronal activity promotes glioma growth through neuroligin-3 secretion. Cell 2015;161(4):803–16.

57. Bonney PA, Boettcher LB, Burks JD, et al. Rates of seizure freedom after surgical resection of diffuse low-grade gliomas. World Neurosurg 2017;106: 750–6.

58. Englot DJ, Berger MS, Barbaro NM, et al. Predictors of seizure freedom after resection of supratentorial low-grade gliomas. A review. J Neurosurg 2011; 115(2):240–4.

59. Xu DS, Awad A-W, Mehalechko C, et al. An extent of resection threshold for seizure freedom in patients with low-grade gliomas. J Neurosurg 2018;128(4): 1084–90.

60. Yordanova YN, Moritz-Gasser S, Duffau H. Awake surgery for WHO Grade II gliomas within "nonelo-quent" areas in the left dominant hemisphere: toward a "supratotal" resection. Clinical article. J Neurosurg 2011;115(2):232–9.

61. Duffau H. Long-term outcomes after supratotal resection of diffuse low-grade gliomas: a consecutive series with 11-year follow-up. Acta Neurochir (Wien) 2016;158(1):51–8.

62. Taillandier L, Duffau H. Epilepsy and insular grade II gliomas: an interdisciplinary point of view from a retrospective monocentric series of 46 cases. Neurosurg Focus 2009;27(2):E8.

63. Wang DD, Deng H, Hervey-Jumper SL, et al. Seizure outcome after surgical resection of insular glioma. Neurosurgery 2017;47(4):175.

64. Blonski M, Taillandier L, Herbet G, et al. Combination of neoadjuvant chemotherapy followed by surgical resection as a new strategy for WHO grade II gliomas: a study of cognitive status and quality of life. J Neurooncol 2011;106(2):353–66.

65. Blonski M, Pallud J, Gozé C, et al. Neoadjuvant chemotherapy may optimize the extent of resection of World Health Organization grade II gliomas: a case series of 17 patients. J Neurooncol 2013; 113(2):267–75.

66. Neal A, Kwan P, O'Brien TJ, et al. IDH1 and IDH2 mutations in postoperative diffuse glioma-associated epilepsy. Epilepsy Behav 2018;78:30–6.

67. van den Bent MJ, Afra D, de Witte O, et al. Long-term efficacy of early versus delayed radiotherapy for low-grade astrocytoma and oligodendroglioma in adults: the EORTC 22845 randomised trial. Lancet 2005;366(9490):985–90.

68. Kiebert GM, Curran D, Aaronson NK, et al. Quality of life after radiation therapy of cerebral low-grade gliomas of the adult: results of a randomised phase III trial on dose response (EORTC trial 22844). EORTC radiotherapy co-operative group. Eur J Cancer 1998;34(12):1902–9.

69. Klein M, Engelberts NHJ, van der Ploeg HM, et al. Epilepsy in low-grade gliomas: the impact on cognitive function and quality of life. Ann Neurol 2003; 54(4):514–20.

70. Eseonu CI, Rincon-Torroella J, Lee YM, et al. Intraoperative seizures in awake craniotomy for perirolandic glioma resections that undergo cortical mapping. J Neurol Surg A Cent Eur Neurosurg 2018;79(3):239–46.

71. Pallud J, Varlet P, Devaux B, et al. Diffuse low-grade oligodendrogliomas extend beyond MRI-defined abnormalities. Neurology 2010;74(21):1724–31.

72. Martino J, Taillandier L, Moritz-Gasser S, et al. Reoperation is a safe and effective therapeutic strategy in recurrent WHO grade II gliomas within eloquent areas. Acta Neurochir (Wien) 2009;151(5):427–36 [discussion: 436].

73. Peeters S, Pagès M, Gauchotte G, et al. Interactions between glioma and pregnancy: insight from a 52-case multicenter series. J Neurosurg 2018;128(1): 3–13.

74. Pallud J, Mandonnet E, Deroulers C, et al. Pregnancy increases the growth rates of World Health Organization grade II gliomas. Ann Neurol 2010; 67(3):398–404.

75. Ruda R, Magliola U, Bertero L, et al. Seizure control following radiotherapy in patients with diffuse gliomas: a retrospective study. Neuro Oncol 2013; 15(12):1739–49.

76. Pallud J, Llitjos J-F, Dhermain F, et al. Dynamic imaging response following radiation therapy predicts long-term outcomes for diffuse low-grade gliomas. Neuro Oncol 2012;14(4):496–505.

77. Brada M, Viviers L, Abson C, et al. Phase II study of primary temozolomide chemotherapy in patients with WHO grade II gliomas. Ann Oncol 2003; 14(12):1715–21.

78. Ngo L, Nei M, Glass J. Temozolomide treatment of refractory epilepsy in a patient with an oligodendroglioma. Epilepsia 2006;47(7):1237–8.

79. Pace A, Vidiri A, Galiè E, et al. Temozolomide chemotherapy for progressive low-grade glioma: clinical benefits and radiological response. Ann Oncol 2003;14(12):1722–6.

80. Sherman JH, Moldovan K, Yeoh HK, et al. Impact of temozolomide chemotherapy on seizure frequency in patients with low-grade gliomas. J Neurosurg 2011;114(6):1617–21.

81. Koekkoek JAF, Dirven L, Heimans JJ, et al. Seizure reduction is a prognostic marker in low-grade glioma patients treated with temozolomide. J Neurooncol 2015;126(2):347–54.

82. Frenay MP, Fontaine D, Vandenbos F, et al. First-line nitrosourea-based chemotherapy in symptomatic non-resectable supratentorial pure low-grade astrocytomas. Eur J Neurol 2005;12(9):685–90.

83. Lebrun C, Fontaine D, Bourg V, et al. Treatment of newly diagnosed symptomatic pure low-grade oligodendrogliomas with PCV chemotherapy. Eur J Neurol 2007;14(4):391–8.

84. Di Bonaventura C, Albini M, D'Elia A, et al. Epileptic seizures heralding a relapse in high grade gliomas. Seizure 2017;51:157–62.

85. Avila EK, Chamberlain M, Schiff D, et al. Seizure control as a new metric in assessing efficacy of tumor treatment in low-grade glioma trials. Neuro Oncol 2017;19(1):12–21.

Treatment

Treatment

Mapping in Low-Grade Glioma Surgery
Low- and High-Frequency Stimulation

Marco Rossi, MD[a,b,1], Sepehr Sani, MD[c,1],
Marco Conti Nibali, MD[a,b], Luca Fornia, PhD[d],
Lorenzo Bello, MD[a,b,2,*], Richard W. Byrne, MD[c,2]

KEYWORDS

- Low-grade glioma • Brain mapping • Low-frequency stimulation • High-frequency stimulation

KEY POINTS

- Surgery for lower grade gliomas aimed at maximal tumor resection, associated with full patient functional integrity.
- Full patient functional integrity is accomplished during resection by the use of brain mapping techniques.
- Brain mapping techniques refers to a group of techniques that allow safe and effective removal of tumor infiltration, generally located in the so-called eloquent or functional areas, preserving the functional integrity of the patients.

INTRODUCTION

Surgery for lower grade gliomas (LGGs) aimed at maximal tumor resection, associated with full patient functional integrity. This goal is accomplished during resection by the use of brain mapping techniques. This term refers to a group of techniques, which allow to safely and effectively remove tumor infiltration, generally located in so-called eloquent or functional areas, preserving the functional integrity of the patients.

The concept of detecting and preserving the essential functional cortical and subcortical sites has been recently defined as surgery according to functional boundaries, and it is summarized with the term functional neuroncologic approach.

The shift of the paradigm between image-based surgery and surgery based on functions finds its rationale on various considerations. (1) Most LGGs are located in areas of the brain traditionally defined as eloquent (language, motor); therefore, resection of tumors within these areas has to be necessarily associated with function preservations. (2) LGGs are highly infiltrative tumors, in which cells could be found beyond the borders of the tumors as visualized in fluid attenuation inversion recovery images, which makes approaches based to pure images quite limited in

Disclosure: Dr Bello was supported by AIRC grant number 18482.
[a] Unit of Neurosurgical Oncology, Department of Hematology and Hemato–Oncology Università degli Studi di Milano, Via Manzoni 56, 20089 Rozzano (MI), Italy; [b] Neurosurgical Oncology, Humanitas Research Hospital, IRCCS, Via Manzoni 56, 20089 Rozzano (MI), Italy; [c] Department of Neurosurgery, Rush University Medical Center, 600 S Paulina Street, Chicago, IL 60612, USA; [d] Laboratory of Motor Control, Department of Medical Biotechnologies and Translational Medicine, Università degli Studi di Milano, Humanitas Research Hospital, IRCCS, Milano 20089, Italy
[1] Dr Marco Rossi and Dr Sepehr Sani share first authorship.
[2] Dr Richard W. Byrne and Dr Lorenzo Bello share last authorship.
* Corresponding author. Unit of Neurosurgical Oncology, Department of Hematology and Hemato-Oncology Università degli Studi di Milano, Via Manzoni 56, 20089 Rozzano (MI), Italy.
E-mail address: lorenzo.bello@unimi.it

term of oncologic results. (3) LGGs are characterized by a slow speed of growth, which induces a progressive reorganization of surrounding brain areas, modifying and reshaping brain functional organization in a way that is patient specific and that cannot be fully depicted by functional images techniques (eg, functional MRI).[1–3] The functional approach exploits the functional reorganization reached by patient brain, allowing the removal of as much tumor as is feasible, possibly extending resection far beyond the visible tumor margins and detectable by conventional MRIs, and preserving functional integrity. The new paradigm (or philosophy) stands in looking for functional brain boundaries independently from where they are located with respect to tumor borders, continuing resection until they are encountered.

Brain mapping techniques include intraoperative neurophysiology and neuropsychology. Intraoperative neurophysiology consists of mapping and monitoring tools. In this article, we discuss indications for the use of brain mapping techniques for LGGs. Within the mapping and monitoring techniques, we focus on the use of low- and high-frequency (HF) stimulation.

INDICATIONS

In the traditional approach, LGGs location is reviewed on preoperative MRI and classified into 3 groups: eloquent, near-eloquent, and noneloquent. Topographic regions of the brain presumed eloquent[4–6] include the primary sensorimotor cortices, dominant posterior superior temporal gyrus, and the inferior parietal lobule, dominant frontal operculum, calcarine visual cortex, basal ganglia, internal capsule, thalamus, and subcortical white matter pathways of each hemisphere. If any part of the lesion is found to infiltrate these regions, it is regarded as being located in an eloquent region; if it approaches, but does not clearly involve these regions, it is considered near-eloquent, and if it is situated in a separate anatomic location it is considered noneloquent. Consequently, LGG located in eloquent and near-eloquent brain areas were those that were considered for surgery with stimulation mapping.

However, considering that, in the functional neurooncologic approach, resection for LGGs should be performed looking for functional boundaries in all cases, the use of brain mapping techniques is always recommended, independent of tumor location. The surgeon must have in his or her mind the architecture of the functional map of the networks surrounding the tumor, adopting and varying the tests to be performed during the intraoperative mapping, to identify and recognize each boundary

during the various stages of the procedure. If the patient is being considered for an awake craniotomy with mapping, such as for most of the cases, strong consideration must be given to the patient's baseline dysphasia, confusion, and anxiety as well as the ability to tolerate an awake craniotomy. **Box 1** provides a list of what are traditionally considered contraindications to awake craniotomy. In these cases, the use of advanced intraoperative neurophysiologic techniques or the use of short awake phase may be of some help.

PREOPERATIVE BRAIN MAPPING PREPARATION

A thorough understanding of the patient's baseline cognitive and language function is paramount, because it provides mandatory information of the level of functional reorganization reached by the patient's brain and is used in performing the resection. This process aids both the surgeon and patient in developing a surgical plan on the extent of resection and reducing or avoiding postoperative permanent deficits.[7,8] Formal neuropsychological evaluations is, therefore, mandatory and not only reserved for lesions involving or is near the language network. Often there are "silent" deficits present preoperatively that may go unnoticed.[9,10]

A detailed presurgical rehearsal and review of expectations during the awake portion of the operation can be very helpful in allaying patient anxiety and ensuring a cooperative patient. If language mapping is anticipated, extensive presurgical counseling is provided on the nature of intraoperative testing. Different tests are administered, targeted, and normalized to population and spoken language. Ideally, all functional domains (memory, language, praxis, executive functions, and fluid intelligence) should be assessed to give a comprehensive map of the degree of functional reorganization reached by the individual patient brain. The surgeon must then proceed toward the design of the detailed surgical procedure that has to be tailored to the individual case and needs.

Box 1
Relative contraindications for awake craniotomy

- Uncooperative patient
- Pediatrics (<10 years old)
- Extreme obesity
- Airway concerns
- Extreme mass effect (consider staging)
- Significant dysphasia

SURGICAL CONSIDERATIONS
Neuroanesthesia

For general anesthesia, a routine cranial neuroa-nesthesia protocol is followed. In awake crani-otomy cases, different regimens can be used: total awake, asleep–awake, and asleep–awake–asleep. In asleep–awake and asleep–awake–asleep cases, a laryngeal mask is used to ensure patient ventilation. Generally, before the incision is made, midazolam (2 mg; avoided if an electro-encephalogram is to be recorded) and fentanyl (50–100 µg) are administered. During surgery, either propofol (50–100 µg/kg of body weight per minute; avoided if an electroencephalogram is to be recorded) or dexmedetomidine (0.2–.7 µg/kg/h) and remifentanil (0.05–0.2 µg/kg/min) are given. Once the craniotomy is performed, the dura is anesthetized along either side of the middle meningeal artery. Anesthetic agents are discontin-ued after the dura is opened.

Craniotomy

A localized craniotomy is performed using a stan-dard neurosurgical technique with the eventual assistance of neuronavigation or other available imaging techniques. A tailored craniotomy is preferred, including the underlying lesion, along with exposure of adjacent functional landmarks. Ideally, the patient awakens as the dura is opened. Pain upon awakening can be addressed with local anesthetic. Often pain is related to the temporalis muscle, which is difficult to block. Releasing trac-tion on the muscle can relieve pain.

STIMULATION MAPPING

Two stimulation paradigms are available: low-frequency (also called bipolar stimulation or Pen-field technique) and HF stimulation.

THE USE OF BIPOLAR STIMULATION

Bipolar stimulation is the traditional method of brain stimulation originally described by Fritsch and Hitzig.[11] Since then, significant experience with this technique has shown its efficacy in cortical and subcortical mapping, particularly around the motor and language cortices. The bi-polar probe has 2 tips separated by 6 to 10 mm (**Fig. 1**). The charge density is focused primarily between the poles, creating a homogenous elec-tric field that is nearly parallel between the tips. When compared with monopolar stimulation, the bipolar technique provides a higher resolution map of the surface being stimulated. Bipolar stim-ulation is more time consuming because it requires manual stimulation before, and in series, with microsurgical resection, but continuous moni-toring during resection is not possible. Bipolar stimulation is also limited in stimulating deeper subcortical structures through the pial surface when compared with monopolar stimulation.

Equipment

The following is a listing of the standard material and equipment used for cortical and subcortical brain mapping during resection operation:

a. Electrocorticography monitoring by placement of an electrode strip or grid on the cortical sur-face to monitor after-discharges (not used by all teams worldwide).
b. Electroencephalogram cables and strips or grids.
c. Cortical stimulation probe and box with power source verified (eg, Ojemann Cortical Stimu-lator [Radionics Corp., Burlington, MA] or another commercially available probe).
d. Counted and linked map tags for cortical iden-tification during mapping.

A B

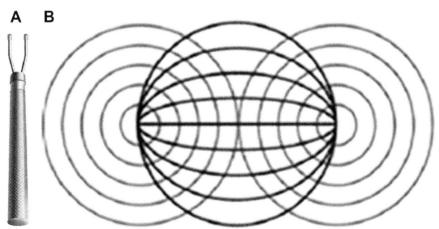

Fig. 1. Bipolar stimulation equipment and charge density. (*A*) Figurative representation of a typical bipolar stim-ulating electrode. (*B*) Charge field density representation of bipolar stimulation.

e. Cold saline or Ringer's solution for irrigation to abrogate an induced seizure during stimulation.
f. Neuropsychological assessment team with naming cards for speech mapping.
g. Dedicated and experienced neuroanesthesiologist.

Sensorimotor Stimulation

Cortical mapping begins by stimulating the temporalis muscle, if exposed, to ensure visual muscle contraction. If no contraction is seen up to 10 mA of stimulation, a systemic check is done (cable connections, paralytic levels, stimulation parameters, battery, etc). We recommend the use of a bipolar probe with 2 tips separated by 7 to 10 mm for optimal stimulation of the cortical pyramidal tracts. The probe is placed on the pial surface, adjacent and parallel to the sulcus.

Bipolar stimulation parameters are summarized in **Table 1**. We prefer motor mapping before language mapping. Initial parameters include 1 to 2 mA, with a frequency of 60 Hz and a pulse duration of 1 ms are used. Cortical patches of 1 cm^3 are stimulated sequentially with rest periods between stimulations. The probe is applied to the cortex for 3 seconds and motor contractions or electromyographic changes (for motor mapping) or reporting of onset and location of any perceived paresthesias by patient (for sensory mapping) are noted. Stimulation starts in the suprasylvian portion of the motor or sensory gyri and advanced superiorly, thereby sequentially identifying the tongue, lip, and hand areas. If the operation is being performed under general anesthesia, only motor mapping is possible.[5] Stimulation parameters remain the same, but usually a higher threshold of initial stimulation is used (3–6 mA). Stimulation intensity increases until contralateral movement is observed by the anesthesiologist or the examiner; alternatively, the detection of responses is also possible. Amplitudes of greater than 10 mA are not recommended in motor cortex stimulation. Stimulating different areas in sequence rather that immediately adjacent areas and using pauses

of at least 10 seconds between stimulations decreases the risk of intraoperative seizures (**Fig. 2**).

Language Mapping

Language mapping is done in the awake patient when the lesion involves the dominant perisylvian frontotemporal region or the subcortical white matter tracts. Intraoperative language mapping is not useful in patients with significant language deficits. Mapping is initiated at stimulation parameters of 1.5 to 3 mA, a frequency of 50 to 60 Hz, and a pulse duration of 1 ms. Once identified, cortical patches of 5 mm are stimulated sequentially with rest periods between stimulations. The probe is applied to the cortex for 1 to 3 seconds and the patient is monitored. Each cortical patch is tested up to 3 times. Electrocorticography may be monitored for afterdischarges, because they can produce false localizing results during mapping and may lead to a clinical seizure. For each site, the patient is tested for counting errors, object naming errors, and word reading errors as they are presented on naming cards. A cortical area is considered positive for language function if the patient is unable to count, name objects, repeat words, or read words in 2 out of 3 stimulations.[12] Speech arrest can be attributed to a stimulus disturbance of language function or arrest of motor activity. Indeed, a combined language and motor function in these cortical areas has been suggested.[13] All positive language areas, vascular supplies, and white matter connections must be preserved during resection (**Fig. 3**).[14,15]

Subcortical Stimulation Mapping

Bipolar stimulation is used to identify subcortical U, association, and projection fibers. Stimulation parameters are generally similar to cortical mapping but higher amplitudes can be needed. Once thresholds for motor activation are identified, repeated stimulations are done as resection progresses. Fiber activation thresholds can be skewed owing to vasogenic edema and mechanical compression by LGG. Thus, obtaining a baseline threshold of activation is key and will serve as a comparison for repeated measures (**Figs. 4** and **5**).

Bipolar Stimulation Pitfalls

Bipolar stimulation necessitates 2 to 4 seconds of manual stimulation by the surgeon, which can be time consuming and disruptive to the flow of LGG resection, particularly during subcortical resection. Continuous stimulation is not possible with bipolar stimulation, explaining why continuous cognitive monitoring is recommended throughout the resection. In the premotor frontal

Table 1
Bipolar stimulation parameters

	Bipolar Settings
Intensity	1–6 mA
Frequency	50–60 Hz
Duration	2–4 s
Filter	10 Hz – 10 kHz
Sensitivity	50–100 µV/Div

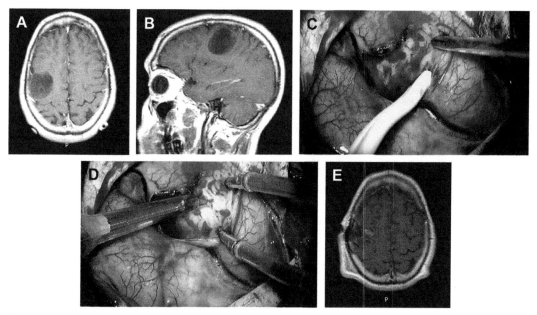

Fig. 2. A 42-year-old right-handed man presented with new-onset focal seizures. Examination was nonrevealing. MRI of brain revealed a low attenuation lesion involving the right supplementary motor, perisylvian region (*A, B*). Bipolar stimulation during awake surgery identified the central sulcus and primary motor strip. Cortical resection ensued, followed by subcortical bipolar stimulation of corticospinal tract (*C, D*) to ensure preservation during posterior wall resection of the tumor. Postoperatively, transient mild left hand weakness was noted, which resolved in follow-up. Postoperative MRI (*E*) revealed total resection.

cortex, bipolar stimulation is more sensitive in localizing the functional area.

Summary Algorithm

A summary of steps for surgical planning and brain mapping during LGG surgery is provided in **Fig. 4**.

THE USE OF HIGH-FREQUENCY STIMULATION MAPPING

The train of pulses HF technique was introduced by Taniguchi in 1993[16] as a monitoring technique. The stimulus has a monophasic form, a duration of 0.5 ms, and it can be administered as a train of stimuli (generally 5, train of 5) separated by 4 ms (the interstimulus interval), and delivered every 1 s (repetition rate 1 Hz) or every 2 s (repetition rate 0.5 Hz). The HF is generally delivered with a monopolar probe, toward to a reference electrode; less frequently, it can be delivered by a bipolar probe that provides more focal stimulation.[17]

Use of High Frequency for Motor Mapping

When HF is applied over the primary motor cortex, usually delivered by a monopolar probe, the response evoked by HF is a motor evoked potential (MEP) and needs a electromyography machine to

be recorded. MEP provides both qualitative (type or group of muscle evoked; **Figs. 2**, **3** and **5**A) and quantitative parameters (MEP amplitude, latency, current intensity; **Fig. 5**B, D) to be used for response interpretation. A fundamental concept during stimulation is the identification at each site of the threshold of motor stimulation, that is, the identification of the lowest current intensity that evokes at the point of stimulation, the smallest detectable motor response visible on electromyography (**Fig. 5**C). The stimulation threshold must be identified both at the cortical and the subcortical levels. At the cortical level, it helps in evaluating the level of excitability of the primary motor cortex, which gives insight on the well-being status of the motor system (for hand muscle responses, generally 3–7 mA in the awake patient; 9–12 mA in the asleep patient when the HF is used), and at the subcortical level, it allows an evaluation of the distance from the motor fibers. In the case of the use of HF, there is a relationship between the amount of current delivered by the stimulator and the distance from the motor tract (1 mA of current used for stimulation and 1 mm of distance from the corticospinal tract; 1 mA – 1 mm rule). A subcortical stimulation threshold of 3 to 5 mA is the minimum recommended to achieve a safe resection and not to endanger the motor tract. HF is considered

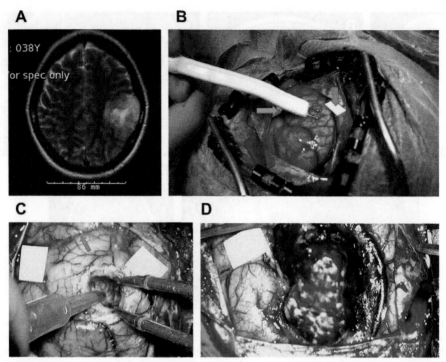

Fig. 3. A 38-year-old right-handed woman with new onset focal seizures. Examination was nonrevealing. Neuro-psychological and language evaluation were without deficits. MRI of the brain revealed a left-sided nonenhancing lesion involving the perisylvian primary sensorimotor region (*A*). functional MRI was consistent with left-sided language organization. Bipolar cortical stimulation during awake mapping identified the face sensory area (*blue arrow, B*) and language positive area (*green arrow, B*). Resection ensued in the least eloquent area and proceeded to sensory then language areas, from sulcus to sulcus followed by deeper resection adjacent to deep white matter pathways of the superior longitudinal fasciculus and arcuate fasciculus (*C; blue arrow,* sylvian fissure). The extent of resection is shown in (*D*). The resection cavity is seen bypassing the white matter, postcentral sulcus, sylvian fissure, and to the area of positive speech arrest.

the most efficient stimulation paradigm for investigating the motor cortex and originating fibers. HF (train of stimuli) is in fact applicable to most tumors, even in the presence of high infiltration of the motor pathways, marked motor pathways compression, a history of uncontrolled seizures, or previous treatments. Furthermore, stimulation is not influenced by the simultaneous use of an ultrasonic aspirator. In the case of tumors in which the motor pathways are difficult to stimulate, it is possible to change some of the parameters of stimulation (eg, the number of stimuli or the amplitude of the single stimulus), allowing to obtain a motor response in most cases, reducing the cases in which a mapping is not obtained, and avoiding the case of negative mapping. HF is also associated with a decreased incidence of stimulation-induced seizures.

Investigating Nonprimary Motor Areas

Although stimulation of the primary motor cortex and of the its originating fibers can be performed while the patient is in resting condition (either asleep or awake), the identification of motor responses originating from other motor areas and pathways (ventral premotor, or supplementary, parietal) requires the patient's collaboration (awake setting) and the use of appropriate tests for investigating the functional properties of each areas. Both LF and HF stimulation can be applied; HF parameters are discussed elsewhere in this article. The role of nonprimary motor areas in human is not completely clear, but extending the resection in these areas can results in long-term postoperative deficit, such as apraxia with a negative impact on quality of life, as demonstrate in an article recently published by our group.[18] The impact of an uncontrolled resection is such areas has been poorly evaluated in the past and only a few investigations take in account this critical aspect of motor mapping. The most common intraoperative test is a simple movement of the contralateral upper limb.[19] The stimulation of areas and subcortical tracts involved in motor control interfere with the

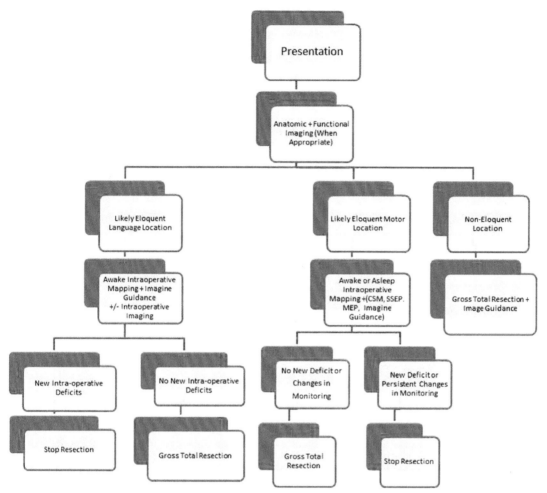

Fig. 4. Treatment paradigm for patients with low-grade glioma and brain mapping planning. CSM, cortical stimulation mapping; MEP, motor evoked potential; SSEP, somatosensory evoked potentials.

ongoing movement. A second, more sensitive and specific test has been recently developed and introduced in clinical routine by our group, namely, the screwdriver test. This test allows to explore in an ecological setting, hand–object integration and provides a better outcome in terms of the preservation of skilled hand movement. During the test, the patient has to perform a rotational movement of a tool that resembles a screwdriver. The stimulation by the mean of direct electrical stimulation (DES) disrupts the ongoing movement, allowing the surgeon to recognize and to preserve brain structure involved in motor control. The application of the test in surgery of glial tumor located 2 cm from the central sulcus has been proved to improve the functional outcome in terms of postoperative hand apraxia. In comparison with the standard test (opening–closing of the hand) the screwdriver test explores hand–object

interaction and allows an evaluation of the role of haptic feedback during hand skilled movement.

Use of High Frequency for Language and Cognitive Mapping

HF stimulation can be applied for both language and cognitive mapping, changing the repetition rate from 1 to 3 Hz. In this case, HF is delivered by a monopolar probe. The current intensity needed to elicit interferences during cognitive or language tasks is usually higher than that required to induce similar responses in the same sites by LF stimulation (close to the double). The use of HF stimulation for cognitive or language mapping is recommended in cases in which LF stimulation (the gold standard) is not properly working (absence of responses even at high current intensity, onset of afterdischarges or seizures). These

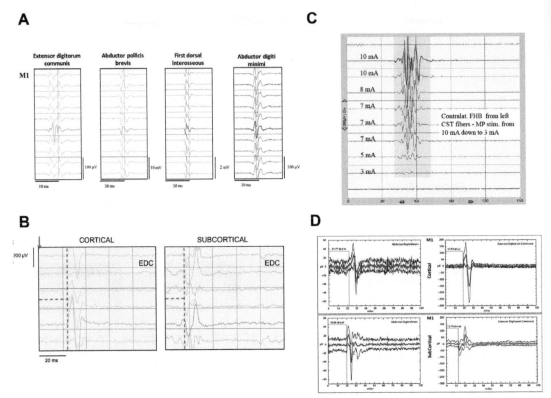

Fig. 5. High-frequency (HF) stimulation for motor mapping. When HF stimulation delivered by a monopolar probe is applied over the primary motor cortex, motor evoked potentials (MEPs), detected by electromyography (EMG), are induced in different muscles, according to primary motor cortex somatotopy (qualitative response) (*A*). HF provides quantitative parameters of the motor response such as latency (*B*, *dotted line*) of the response (*B*, *blue line*) from the stimulus onset (*B*, *blue arrow*); the latency decreases at the subcortical level (*B*). MEP amplitude (*D*) could be also evaluated, both for cortical or subcortical stimulation. The amplitude of MEP response is more variable when is recorded in awake patient (*left*), and it is more stable when the patient is under asleep anesthesia (*right*). A fundamental concept during stimulation is the identification at each site of the threshold of motor stimulation, that is, the identification of the lowest current intensity that evokes at the point of stimulation, the smallest detectable motor response visible on EMG (*C*); this provides information of the distance between the site of the stimulation and M1 originating fibers. CST, corticospinal tract; EDC, extensor digitorium communis; FHB, flexor hallucis brevis.

cases are characterized by a long seizure history, poor controlled seizures, uptake of high dosage of antiepileptic drugs, previous treatments (surgery, radiotherapy, or chemotherapy). The use of HF in these cases allows mapping, extending the benefit of using brain mapping techniques in this difficult subset of patients.[20]

High-Frequency Stimulation for Motor Pathways Monitoring

As previously reported, HF stimulation technique has been developed and introduced in neurosurgery as a monitoring tool.[16] Indeed, the same stimulation paradigm can be applied with a cortical strip placed on the primary motor areas to elicit continuous MEPs through all phases of surgery. Stimulation parameters are the same as

described for standard monopolar motor mapping.[21]

This system is an effective way to monitoring the activity of motor pathways (from the cortex to the effector) and it is sensitive for any vascular damage. This method is particularly useful during resection of deep-seated lesion with a close relationship with vascular structures (ie, insular glioma and anterior perforating arteries).

Any changes of MEPs is reported by the neurophysiologist to the surgeon, who can initiate maneuvers (such as irrigation of the vessels and increasing the mean arterial pressure) trying to obtain a recovery of the MEPs and thus avoiding vascular damage.

Several works have been published seeking to identify a reliable warning criterion in term of percentage of amplitude reduction, but there is no wide consensus.[21] In our opinion, any decrease of MEPs has to be evaluated according to the surgical situation: if a clear correlation with the surgical action exist (ie, MEP reduction during manipulation of critical vessels), any reduction of MEPs has to be taken in account, interrupt the resection for a while, and come back to the critical area later.

SUMMARY

Surgery for LGG requires the use of brain mapping techniques to identify functional boundaries that represent the limit of the resection. Two stimulation paradigms are current available and their use should be tailored to the clinical context to extend tumor removal and decrease the odds of permanent postoperative deficits.

REFERENCES

1. Duffau H, Capelle L. Preferential brain locations of low-grade gliomas: comparison with glioblastomas and review of hypothesis. Cancer 2004;100(12): 2622–6.
2. Wunderlich G, Knorr U, Herzog H, et al. Precentral glioma location determines the displacement of cortical hand representation. Neurosurgery 1998; 42(1):18–26 [discussion 26–7].
3. Duffau H, Denvil D, Capelle L. Long term reshaping of language, sensory, and motor maps after glioma resection: a new parameter to integrate in the surgical strategy. J Neurol Neurosurg Psychiatry 2002; 72(4):511–6.
4. Chang EF, Clark A, Smith Justin S, et al. Functional mapping–guided resection of low-grade gliomas in eloquent areas of the brain: improvement of long-term survival. J Neurosurg 2011;114(3):566–73.
5. Berger MS. Lesions in functional ("eloquent") cortex and subcortical white matter. Clin Neurosurg 1994; 41:444–63.
6. Kim Stefan S, McCutcheon Ian E, Suki D, et al. Awake craniotomy for brain tumors near eloquent cortex. Neurosurgery 2009;64(5):836–46.
7. Satoer D, Visch-Brink E, Smits M, et al. Long-term evaluation of cognition after glioma surgery in eloquent areas. J Neurooncol 2014;116(1):153–60.
8. Satoer D, Vork J, Visch-Brink E, et al. Cognitive functioning early after surgery of gliomas in eloquent areas. J Neurosurg 2012;117(5):831–8.
9. Racine Caroline A, Li J, Molinaro Annette M, et al. Neurocognitive function in newly diagnosed low-grade glioma patients undergoing surgical resection with awake mapping techniques. Neurosurgery 2015;77(3):371–9.
10. Rostomily RC, Keles GE, Berger MS. Radical surgery in the management of low-grade and high-grade gliomas. Baillieres Clin Neurol 1996;5(2): 345–69.
11. Fritsch G, Hitzig E. Electric excitability of the cerebrum (Über die elektrische Erregbarkeit des Grosshirns). Epilepsy Behav 2009;15(2):123–30.
12. Ojemann G, Ojemann J, Lettich E, et al. Cortical language localization in left, dominant hemisphere. J Neurosurg 1989;71(3):316–26.
13. Kimura D. Left-hemisphere control of oral and brachial movements and their relation to communication. Philos Trans R Soc Lond B Biol Sci 1982; 298(1089):135–49.
14. Gil-Robles S, Duffau H. Surgical management of World Health Organization Grade II gliomas in eloquent areas: the necessity of preserving a margin around functional structures. Neurosurg Focus 2010;28(2):E8.
15. Vannemreddy P, Byrne R. Advances and limitations of cerebral cortex functional mapping. Contemp Neurosurg 2011;33(25):1–6.
16. Taniguchi M, Cedzich C, Schramm J. Modification of cortical stimulation for motor evoked potentials under general anesthesia: technical description. Neurosurgery 1993;32(2):219–26.
17. Bello L, Riva M, Fava E, et al. Tailoring neurophysiological strategies with clinical context enhances resection and safety and expands indications in gliomas involving motor pathways. Neuro Oncol 2014; 16(8):1110–28.
18. Rossi M, Fornia L, Puglisi G, et al. Assessment of the praxis circuit in glioma surgery to reduce the incidence of postoperative and long-term apraxia: a new intraoperative test. J Neurosurg 2018;1–11. https://doi.org/10.3171/2017.7.JNS17357.
19. Braem B, Honoré J, Rousseaux M, et al. Integration of visual and haptic informations in the perception of the vertical in young and old healthy adults and right brain-damaged patients. Neurophysiol Clin 2014; 44(1):41–8.
20. Riva M, Fava E, Gallucci M, et al. Monopolar high-frequency language mapping: can it help in the surgical management of gliomas? A comparative clinical study. J Neurosurg 2016;124(5):1479–89.
21. MacDonald DB, Skinner S, Shils J, et al. Intraoperative motor evoked potential monitoring – A position statement by the American Society of Neurophysiological Monitoring. Clin Neurophysiol 2013;124(12): 2291–316.

Surgical Adjuncts to Increase the Extent of Resection
Intraoperative MRI, Fluorescence, and Raman Histology

Todd Hollon, MD[a], Walter Stummer, Prof Dr Med[b],
Daniel Orringer, MD[a], Eric Suero Molina, MBA, Dr Med[b,*]

KEYWORDS

- Low-grade glioma • Fluorescence-guided resections • 5-Aminolevulnic acid • Intraoperative MRI
- Raman spectroscopy • Stimulated Raman histology

KEY POINTS

- Intraoperative MRI increases the extent of resection in both low-grade and high-grade gliomas.
- Approximately 20% of low-grade gliomas will demonstrate 5-aminolevulinic acid (5-ALA)-induced protoporphyrin IX fluorescence.
- Fluorescence-guidance with 5-ALA can assist in finding anaplastic foci in low-grade tumors and provide accurate adjuvant treatment.
- Raman spectroscopy can detect viable tumor in brain biopsy specimens and identify brain tumor infiltration in vivo.
- Coherent Raman scattering microscopy provides label-free histologic images and can assist intraoperative brain tumor diagnosis.

INTRODUCTION

Surgery is the first step in a multimodal therapy for malignant glioma. The extent of resection is a key surgical outcome for reducing the rate of recurrence and maximizing overall and progression-free survival in high-grade[1–7] and low-grade glioma (LGG).[8,9] However, it is well known that tumor margins, due to their infiltrative growth, are difficult to depict and neither macroscopically perceptive nor tangible to surgeons' hands or instruments. In a landmark paper in 1994, Albert and colleagues[10] demonstrated, by performing early postoperative MRI, how surgeons strongly underestimate residual tumor when solely relying on visual and tactical senses. The introduction of surgical tools; for example, neuronavigation in the early 1990s, improved the surgeons' orientation during surgery and helped tailor approaches and reduce the size of craniotomies.[11] However, brain-shift after dura opening and throughout tumor resection limits its value as surgery is performed.[12,13] Further surgical tools are emerging to assist neurosurgeons. This article outlines advantages and provides a comprehensive review

Disclosure Statement: W. Stummer has provided consultant and speakers services to Medac (Wedel), Carl Zeiss (Oberkochen), Leica (Heerburg). T. Hollon has received grant number R01CA226527. The other authors have nothing to disclose.
[a] Department of Neurosurgery, University of Michigan, 1500 East Medical Center Drive, Ann Arbor, MI 48109, USA; [b] Department of Neurosurgery, University Hospital of Münster, Albert-Schweitzer-Campus 1, Geb. A1, Münster 48149, Germany
* Corresponding author.
E-mail address: eric.suero@ukmuenster.de

Neurosurg Clin N Am 30 (2019) 65–74
https://doi.org/10.1016/j.nec.2018.08.012

of surgical adjuncts feasible for maximizing the extent of resection in LGG surgery, that is, intraoperative MRI (iMRI), fluorescence-guided surgery (FGS), and Raman histology.

INTRAOPERATIVE MRI

A limitation of standard frameless stereotactic navigation is a lack of an updated navigational dataset during brain tumor resections. Brain shift related to loss of cerebrospinal fluid, brain dependency, edema, and tumor removal results in stereotactic inaccuracies. iMRI can be used to determine the extent of residual tumor burden and provide updated navigational data. Several studies have shown iMRI to increase the extent of resection in LGG and malignant glioma surgery.[8,14–18] Claus and colleagues[8] conducted a retrospective study evaluating progression-free and overall survival rates for patients who underwent resection of LGGs using iMRI compared with age-adjusted and histology-adjusted controls from a national database. The 1-year, 2-year, and 5-year death rates were 1.9%, 3.6%, and 17.6%, respectively. These results show a significant decrease in death rates when compared with matched controls (10%, 16%, and 29%, respectively).

A randomized, controlled trial was performed to evaluate the efficacy of iMRI for increasing the extent of resection in glioma surgery. Subjects were randomized to either an iMRI-guided arm or a conventional resection with neuronavigation arm.[19] The primary endpoint was the extent of resection, with secondary endpoints of postoperative tumor volume and progression-free survival at 60 months. A total of 49 subjects were included in the data analysis, with 24 subjects in the iMRI group and 25 subjects in the control group. Although 96% of the subjects in the iMRI arm had a complete resection, only 68% of the subjects in the control group had complete resection; this difference was statistically significant for the investigators' primary endpoint. The data did demonstrate that complete resection was a strong predictor of 6-month progression-free survival; however, there was no statistically significant difference in progression-free survival between the 2 study arms. No subject in whom residual tumor was identified intraoperatively and subsequently underwent further resection after scanning developed postoperative neurologic deficits. This indicates that resection of residual tumor identified with iMRI does not expose the patient to additional risk for postoperative neurologic deficits. A review of surgical results did not show iMRI-guided surgery to result in additional neurologic deficits, including cases in which intraoperative imaging resulted in further, more aggressive resection.[20] These findings indicated that iMRI is an important tool for maximizing the extent of resection without exposing patients to additional surgical risk.

Eyupoglu and colleagues[17] noticed that iMRI can help reveal low-grade portions of allegedly secondary glioblastomas and improve the extent of resection. Furthermore, high-field iMRI seems to be superior in LGG surgery[16,18]; Senft and colleagues[21] reported not achieving complete resection in a large portion of analyzed LGG while using a low-field iMRI owing to poor anatomic resolution. In contrast, Hirschl and colleagues[15] described a sensitivity of 82% and specificity of 95% of low-field iMRI, and claimed feasibility for detecting residual tumor in LGG surgery. Nevertheless, impact of overall survival associated with the extent of resection remains debatable.

However, iMRI carries the limitation of being expensive and time-consuming. Implementation will increase surgery by at least 1 hour after performing and evaluating images.[17,19] A further caveat is the leakage of gadolinium contrast into the resection cavity, challenging imaging interpretation.[22]

FLUORESCENCE-GUIDANCE USING 5-AMINOLEVULINIC ACID

Five-aminolevulinic acid (5-ALA) is a heme-precursor that induces synthesis and accumulation of fluorescent protoporphyrin IX (PPIX) in malignant glioma. As such, 5-ALA's clinical value in the surgery of high-grade gliomas is undisputable. After its introduction in 1998[23] and its approval by the European Medicine Agencies after a randomized multicenter phase III trial,[24] FGS with 5-ALA is now used worldwide, having recently been approved by the US Food and Drug Administration. Assisted by commercially available microscopes equipped with specialized filter systems and an excitation light with a wavelength of 405 nm, PPIX fluorescence can be seen in real-time during surgery. 5-ALA is administrated orally 4 hours before surgery at a dose of 20 mg/kg body weight.[25] In the authors' experience, fluorescence maximum occurs 6 to 8 hours after administration.

High-grade glioma surgery with fluorescence-guidance mediated by 5-ALA has become standard in the current neurosurgery era.[22,24–30] So far, it is known that about 20% of LGG fluoresce after 5-ALA administration.[31,32] However, for tumors harboring typical MRI characteristics of LGG, an anaplastic focus can be found in 44% to 55% of cases,[33,34] which can be uncovered using fluoroethyl (FET)-PET tomography. In these cases, fluorescence-guidance can assist in finding these anaplastic foci during surgery, providing tissue for accurate histopathological diagnosis, and assuring adequate grading. Jaber and colleagues[35] evaluated factors for predicting fluorescence in lesions suspicious of LGG. The investigators concluded that age, tumor, volume, and 18F-fluoroethyl-L-thyrosin-(FET)-PET uptake ratio greater than 1.85 significantly correlates with predicting fluorescence. Furthermore, if any sign of contrast-enhancement was apparent in MRI, the probability of intraoperative fluorescence significantly increased.

5-ALA advantages and disadvantages in the context of LGG surgery are listed in **Table 1**. As a body's own metabolite, 5-ALA induces specific PPIX-fluorescence in tumor cells, whereas other agents; for example, fluorescein, as an exogenous fluorophore without any specific affinity to tumor cells, acts more as a blood-brain barrier breakdown marker.[36] Unspecific extravasation of fluorescein has been reported in perifocal edema.[37] A profound understanding and experience is required to discriminate fluorescein from edema propagation or disruption of blood-brain barrier in tumor tissue. Furthermore, time-dependency when using fluorescein, as well as its clinical value when treating LGGs, is poorly studied to date. It is, however, still unclear if fluorescent low-grade tumors represent a more malignant subtype of gliomas with poorer prognosis.

RAMAN HISTOLOGY
Label-Free Tumor Detection

A challenge to iMRI and FGS is the reliance on tumor labeling using an exogenous marker (ie, gadolinium or 5-ALA). Accuracy of tumor labeling can be diminished either by areas containing tumor failing to uptake the exogenous marker (ie, poor sensitivity) or areas without tumor being erroneous labeled (ie, poor specificity).[38] Label-free imaging methods can avoid this challenge by using intrinsic biochemical and histoarchitectural features to differentiate normal brain and tumor tissue. Label-free methods that have been applied to neurosurgical oncology and to the detection of tumor infiltration include mass spectrometry,[39] optical coherence tomography,[40] infrared spectroscopy,[41,42] Raman spectroscopy,[43] coherent anti-Stokes stimulated scattering microscopy,[44] and stimulated Raman scattering (SRS) microscopy.[45] Tumor-infiltrated tissue can produce a unique spectral signature that allows for differentiation from normal brain. This article provides an overview of the application of Raman-based methods for the detection and diagnosis of brain tumors.

Detecting Tumor with Spontaneous Raman Spectroscopy

Raman scattering occurs when the frequency of an incident photon is shifted (increased or decreased) after being scattered by a molecule. This effect is called the Raman shift and underlies all Raman-based imaging methods. A molecule can absorb energy and decrease the scattered photon frequency (Stokes scattering), or can lose energy and increase the photon frequency (anti-Stokes scattering). The Raman shift is relatively weak compared with elastic scattering (ie, Rayleigh scattering, no exchange of energy) and cannot be detected under standard visual conditions. However, using narrow-band laser excitation and spectrometry, Raman spectroscopy can be used to identify molecules and chemical moieties based on signature vibrational frequencies of Raman-active chemical bonds, providing insight into the chemical composition of both inorganic and biological specimens. The biomolecular composition of surgical specimens (eg, protein, lipids, nucleic acids) can produce a unique vibrational fingerprint for both normal brain tissue and brain tumor specimens.

Although the use of Raman spectroscopy to characterize brain tissue dates back to early 1990s,[46] the ability to detect spectral differences between vital tumor and necrotic frozen section specimens from patients with glioblastoma was described in 2002.[47] Necrotic specimens obtained during stereotactic biopsies can have gross appearance similar to vital tumor specimens; however, necrotic specimens often provide insufficient histopathologic information to render a diagnosis. Major spectral difference between necrotic and vital specimens were found due to the high concentrations of cholesterol found in necrotic tissue, allowing for spectral discriminate analysis to accurately classify glioblastoma specimens (**Fig. 1**). Kalkanis and colleagues[48] improved these techniques by developing a 3 Raman channel pseudocolor scheme for intraoperative frozen section labeling.[49,50] Spectral intensities from wavenumber 1004 cm^{-1}, 1300:1344 cm^{-1}, and 1600 cm^{-1} were mapped to a traditional red, green, blue (RGB) color scheme. A color grid of pixel size 300 μm × 300 μm or 2 5 μm × 25 μm was used to visualize spectral differences between normal brain, necrotic tissue, and tumor tissue. Using this method, accuracy for discriminating tissue types was greater than 90% based on the previously listed Raman channels. This technique provided a precedent for using spectral intensities to generate pseudocolor heatmaps to better characterize intraoperative neurosurgical specimens.

In vivo Raman spectroscopy has the added benefit of allowing for spectral analysis of brain tissue in situ. The previously mentioned studies were ex vivo techniques, requiring removal of the tissue before spectra acquisition owing to the limitations

Table 1
Advantages and drawbacks of implantation of the surgical adjuncts discussed in this article during low-grade glioma surgery

	FGS with 5-ALA	iMRI	Raman Histology
Advantages	• Depicts tumor margins • Assists in finding anaplastic foci in low-grade tumors and provides accurate adjuvant treatment • Real-time information direct in the operative field • Fluorescence normally surpasses gadolinium-enhancement • Brain-shift is not an obstacle during surgery • Increases resection rates	• Monitors resection of non-fluorescing and enhancing gliomas • Allows neuronavigation update to overcome brain-shift • 3D imaging overcoming residual tumor in deep brain tissue • Identifies satellite anaplastic lesions • Increases resection rates	• Label-free optical imaging of fresh surgical specimens • Nondestructive technique • Chemical specificity allows for quantitative imaging • Ex vivo and in vivo implementations • Intraoperative digital images allow for computer-aided diagnosis and machine learning
Drawbacks	• ~20% of nonenhancing LGG will fluoresce • Should not be used as single surgical adjunct • Fluorescence can be hidden by blood or healthy tissue • Fluorophore bleaching can occur by light or coagulation	• High cost • Can increase surgery time by ~1 h • Gadolinium can leak intraoperatively, leading to falsely identify healthy tissue • Low-field iMRI probably not as good as high-field iMRI for LGG surgery	• Ideal for small, compressible specimens; difficult-to-image fibrous tumors • Requires specialized optical instrumentation • Ex vivo imaging requires tissue removal

of commercially available Raman spectroscopy systems. More recently, fiberoptic Raman spectroscopy probes have been developed and used intraoperatively for cancer detection. Jermyn and colleagues[43] conducted a clinical study to evaluate the efficacy of a hand-held Raman probe for the intraoperative detecting of tumor infiltration within the resection cavities of LGG and malignant glioma subjects. By analyzing differences in spectral peaks from 400 to 1700 cm^{-1} wavenumbers, tumor-invaded brain (>15% tumor cell infiltration) could be distinguished from normal brain with an accuracy of 92%, sensitivity of 93%, and specificity of 91%. Specimens with tumor infiltration showed differences in lipid bands at 700 (cholesterol) and 1142 (phospholipids) cm^{-1} compared with normal tissue. Hypercellularity within tumor-infiltrated brain resulted in increased spectral intensity at 1540 to 1645 cm^{-1}, corresponding to a higher nucleic acid content. Similar results were found for cerebral brain metastasis.[51] Subsequent clinical studies demonstrated that in vivo Raman spectroscopy was able to detect invasive tumor cells several centimeters beyond pathologic T1-weighted contrast-enhanced and T2-weighted MRI signals.[52] Additionally, a feasibility study found spectral differences between parent glioblastoma and recurrent glioblastoma cells, indicating differential gene expression and underlying biomolecular signatures.[53] These results provide insight into the clinical translation of Raman spectroscopy to improve cancer detection and intraoperative delineation of tumor infiltration.

Coherent Raman Scattering Microscopy for Brain Tumor Imaging

Although spontaneous Raman spectroscopy has high spectral resolution, it is limited by low signal-to-noise ratios, resulting in longer acquisition times and low spatial resolution. Coherent Raman scattering microscopy increases signal intensity over a narrowband spectral region by using 2 excitation beams to coherently drive the vibrational resonance of Raman active chemical bonds. Because coherent Raman scattering produces a signal that is orders of magnitude greater (>10,000 ×) than spontaneous Raman scattering, submicron spatial resolution and video-rate imaging speeds are possible. Two methods of coherent Raman scattering microscopy have been developed and used in biomedical imaging: coherent anti-Stokes Raman scattering (CARS) microscopy and SRS.

CARS was first applied to brain tumor imaging using an orthotopic human astrocytoma mouse model.[54] Ex vivo samples were imaged using 700-μm × 700-μm fields of view to produce

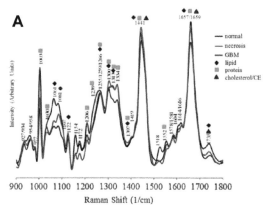

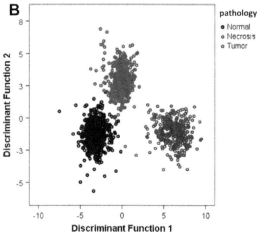

Fig. 1. Raman spectroscopy for discriminating normal brain, necrosis, and tumor tissue. (*A*) Mean spectrum of normal, necrosis, and tumor from training data, with visible Raman peaks labeled. (*B*) Plot of discriminant function analysis scores for training data. CE, cholesterol esters; GBM, glioblastoma. (*From* Kalkanis SN, Kast RE, Rosenblum ML, et al. Raman spectroscopy to distinguish gray matter, necrosis, and glioblastoma multiforme in frozen tissue sections. J Neurooncol 2014;116(3):481; with permission.)

mosaic images of mouse brain coronal sections. Corresponding sections were stained with hematoxylin-eosin (H&E) to confirm concordant histoarchitectural features in CARS images and standard pathologic sections. CARS microscopy was capable of generating chemically sensitive images for lipid (2845 cm^{-1}, hydrocarbon symmetric stretching) and proteins (carbon–hydrogen stretch, 2920 cm^{-1}; amide I vibration, 2960 cm^{-1}) within mouse brain specimens, highlighting lipid-rich myelin and protein-rich tumor cell nuclei, respectively. A similar study was able to identify tumor infiltration in an orthotopic glioblastoma and brain metastasis model using CARS, and results were confirmed in human glioblastoma specimens.[44] To increase the spectral breadth and

chemical sensitivity of CARS, a broadband CARS technique has been developed without compromising imaging speed or sensitivity.[55] The biologically relevant Raman spectral region (500–3500 cm^{-1}) was used to image a xenograft glioblastoma mouse model. Pseudocolor broadband CARS microscopy was able to distinguish white matter, gray matter, and tumor, and to provide nuclear resolution.

SRS microscopy has the advantage of superior nuclear contrast, a linear relationship between signal intensity and chemical concentration, and a nondistorted spectrum nearly identical to spontaneous Raman scattering, making quantitative chemical imaging easier to implement. A landmark paper published in 2008 by Freudiger and colleagues[56] demonstrated the feasibility of label-free biomedical imaging using SRS microscopy. SRS sensitivity to lipid concentration was well-suited for imaging the central nervous system due to the high concentration of lipid-rich myelin. Focusing on the 2845 cm^{-1} shift is ideal for visualizing axon bundles in the corpus callosum due to high lipid content of myelin sheaths. A novel microscope configuration was designed to allow for approximately 30% of the backscattered light to reach the objective, 3 times more than standard microscopy, making in vivo imaging possible. In a subsequent study, Ji and colleagues[57] described SRS microscopy for in vivo label-free imaging of brain tumors. The investigators used video-rate SRS microscopy in combination with a human infiltrative glioblastoma xenograft mouse model. Normal brain and tumor infiltration could be visualized using a cranial window model that allows for direct visualization of the cortical surface. SRS microscopy was able to differentiate normal brain tissue from tumor-infiltrated brain that was indistinguishable on gross appearance. To simulate intraoperative conditions during brain tumor surgery, corticotomy and dissection into the mouse brain was able to yield similar ease of detecting tumor infiltration, with near-perfect concordance ($\kappa = 0.98$) between SRS and H&E microscopy for detection of glioma infiltration based on neuropathologist assessment (**Fig. 2**). Subsequent studies have developed quantitative histologic techniques to automate detection of tumor infiltration and differentiate low-grade versus high-grade tumors.[57,58]

Improvements in fiber-laser technology facilitated the development of a clinical SRS microscope that could be used intraoperatively to image fresh surgical specimens (**Fig. 3**).[45,55,59] Orringer and colleagues[45] imaged fresh surgical specimens from 101 neurosurgical subjects and developed a novel virtual H&E color scheme called

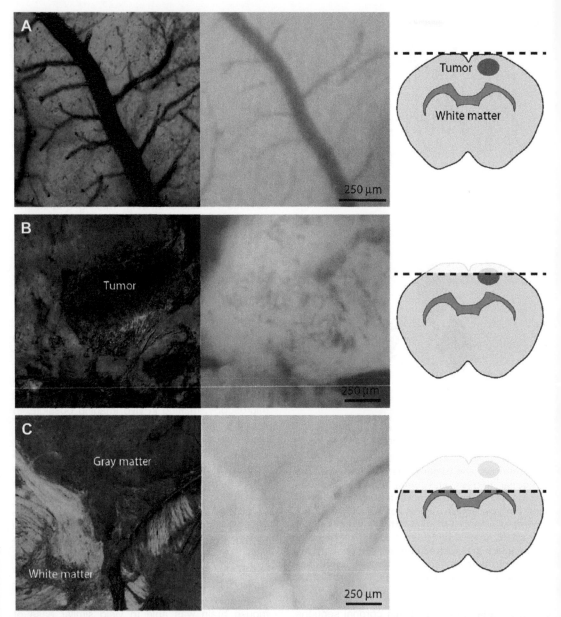

Fig. 2. SRS imaging during simulated tumor resection on a mouse brain. En face, epi-SRS images were obtained in vivo during various stages of a simulated tumor removal. Left column, SRS; middle column; bright-field; right column, depth of imaging. The (*A*) In a tumor located beneath the cortical surface, there is no obvious abnormality in SRS or bright-field images when imaging the cortical surface. (*B*) After a portion of the cortex has been removed, the tumor is revealed. Blood was present on the dissected surface but did not adversely affect the distinction of tumor-infiltrated regions from noninfiltrated regions. (*C*) Because dissection was carried deep past the tumor, the normal appearance of white matter and cortex was again visible. (*From* Ji M, Orringer DA, Freudiger CW, et al. Rapid, label-free detection of brain tumors with stimulated Raman scattering microscopy. Sci Transl Med. 2013;5(201):201ra119; with permission.)

stimulated Raman histology (SRH). Using 30 subjects to simulate an intraoperative pathologic evaluation consultation, near-perfect concordance was found between SRH and conventional histology for predicting diagnosis (Cohen's kappa, $\kappa > 0.89$), with accuracy greater than 92%. The investigators also trained and validated an artificial neural network that predicts brain-tumor subtype with 90% accuracy. Their results provide the first step toward translating SRH to the clinical setting and improve the surgical management of brain tumor patients.

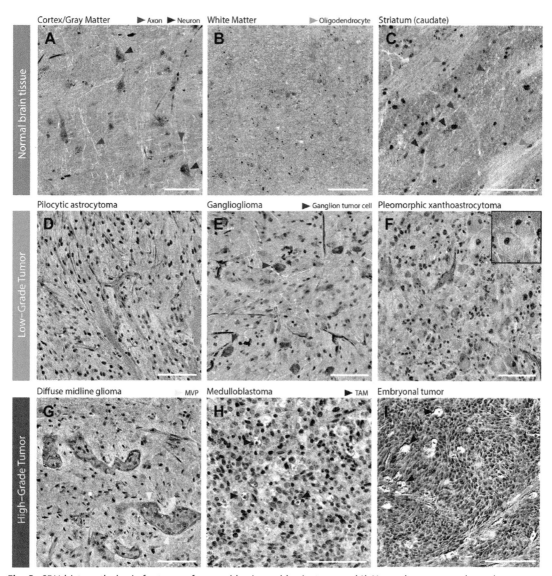

Fig. 3. SRH histopathologic features of normal brain and brain tumors. (*A*) Normal neocortex shows large pyramidal neurons with lipofuscin cytoplasmic inclusions seen in bright pink. Axons are clearly visualized in neocortex as white lines. (*B*) Normal subcortical white matter shows oligodendrocytes embedded in a background of pink, bulbous densely myelinated axons. (*C*) Striatum from a cadaveric specimen shows deep gray matter neurons with striated white matter tracts. (*D*) Pilocytic astrocytoma shows long, delicate piloid glial processes. (*E*) Ganglioglioma has large binucleated ganglion cells in a glial background. (*F*) Pleomorphic xanthoastrocytoma with massive lipidized tumor cells (*insert*). (*G*) Diffuse midline glioma show microvascular proliferation and anaplasia. (*H*) Medulloblastoma and (*I*) other embryonal tumors show hypercellular, small round blue cell morphology and tumor-associated macrophage infiltration. Scale bars are 100 μm. MVP, microvascular proliferation, TAM, tumor-associated macrophage. (*From* Hollon TC, Lewis S, Pandian B, et al. Rapid intraoperative diagnosis of pediatric brain tumors using stimulated Raman histology. Cancer Res 2018;78(1):282; with permission.)

SUMMARY

When available, iMRI significantly increases the extent of resection in LGG. In selected cases, fluorescence-guidance with 5-ALA can provide guidance for maximal resection. 5-ALA administration is recommended if anaplastic foci are suspected; for example, high FET-PET metabolism.

Raman histology is a promising technique that can provide in vivo assistance during surgery.

REFERENCES

1. Kreth FW, Thon N, Simon M, et al. Gross total but not incomplete resection of glioblastoma prolongs

survival in the era of radiochemotherapy. Ann Oncol 2013;24(12):3117–23.

2. Lacroix M, Abi-Said D, Fourney DR, et al. A multivariate analysis of 416 patients with glioblastoma multiforme: prognosis, extent of resection, and survival. J Neurosurg 2001;95(2):190–8.

3. Sanai N, Polley MY, McDermott MW, et al. An extent of resection threshold for newly diagnosed glioblastomas. J Neurosurg 2011;115(1):3–8.

4. Stummer W, Meinel T, Ewelt C, et al. Prospective cohort study of radiotherapy with concomitant and adjuvant temozolomide chemotherapy for glioblastoma patients with no or minimal residual enhancing tumor load after surgery. J Neurooncol 2012;108(1): 89–97.

5. Stummer W, Tonn JC, Mehdorn HM, et al. Counterbalancing risks and gains from extended resections in malignant glioma surgery: a supplemental analysis from the randomized 5-aminolevulinic acid glioma resection study. Clinical article. J Neurosurg 2011;114(3):613–23.

6. Pichlmeier U, Bink A, Schackert G, et al. Resection and survival in glioblastoma multiforme: an RTOG recursive partitioning analysis of ALA study patients. Neuro Oncol 2008;10(6):1025–34.

7. Orringer D, Lau D, Khatri S, et al. Extent of resection in patients with glioblastoma: limiting factors, perception of resectability, and effect on survival. J Neurosurg 2012;117(5):851–9.

8. Claus EB, Horlacher A, Hsu L, et al. Survival rates in patients with low-grade glioma after intraoperative magnetic resonance image guidance. Cancer 2005;103(6):1227–33.

9. Duffau H. Awake surgery for incidental WHO grade II gliomas involving eloquent areas. Acta Neurochir (Wien) 2012;154(4):575–84 [discussion: 584].

10. Albert FK, Forsting M, Sartor K, et al. Early postoperative magnetic resonance imaging after resection of malignant glioma: objective evaluation of residual tumor and its influence on regrowth and prognosis. Neurosurgery 1994;34(1):45–60 [discussion: 60–1].

11. Wadley J, Dorward N, Kitchen N, et al. Pre-operative planning and intra-operative guidance in modern neurosurgery: a review of 300 cases. Ann R Coll Surg Engl 1999;81(4):217–25.

12. Willems PW, van der Sprenkel JW, Tulleken CA, et al. Neuronavigation and surgery of intracerebral tumours. J Neurol 2006;253(9):1123–36.

13. Watts C, Sanai N. Surgical approaches for the gliomas. Handb Clin Neurol 2016;134:51–69.

14. Coburger J, Merkel A, Scherer M, et al. Low-grade glioma surgery in intraoperative magnetic resonance imaging: results of a multicenter retrospective assessment of the German Study Group for intraoperative magnetic resonance imaging. Neurosurgery 2016;78(6):775–86.

15. Hirschl RA, Wilson J, Miller B, et al. The predictive value of low-field strength magnetic resonance imaging for intraoperative residual tumor detection. Clinical article. J Neurosurg 2009;111(2): 252–7.

16. Hatiboglu MA, Weinberg JS, Suki D, et al. Impact of intraoperative high-field magnetic resonance imaging guidance on glioma surgery: a prospective volumetric analysis. Neurosurgery 2009;64(6):1073–81 [discussion: 1081].

17. Eyupoglu IY, Hore N, Savaskan NE, et al. Improving the extent of malignant glioma resection by dual intraoperative visualization approach. PLoS One 2012;7(9):e44885.

18. Tsugu A, Ishizaka H, Mizokami Y, et al. Impact of the combination of 5-aminolevulinic acid-induced fluorescence with intraoperative magnetic resonance imaging-guided surgery for glioma. World Neurosurg 2011;76(1–2):120–7.

19. Senft C, Bink A, Franz K, et al. Intraoperative MRI guidance and extent of resection in glioma surgery: a randomised, controlled trial. Lancet Oncol 2011; 12(11):997–1003.

20. Nimsky C, Fujita A, Ganslandt O, et al. Volumetric assessment of glioma removal by intraoperative high-field magnetic resonance imaging. Neurosurgery 2004;55:358–71.

21. Senft C, Seifert V, Hermann E, et al. Usefulness of intraoperative ultra low-field magnetic resonance imaging in glioma surgery. Neurosurgery 2008;63(4 Suppl 2):257–66 [discussion: 266–7].

22. Suero Molina E, Schipmann S, Stummer W. Maximizing safe resections: the roles of 5-aminolevulinic acid and intraoperative MR imaging in glioma surgery-review of the literature. Neurosurg Rev 2017. [Epub ahead of print].

23. Stummer W, Stocker S, Wagner S, et al. Intraoperative detection of malignant gliomas by 5-aminolevulinic acid-induced porphyrin fluorescence. Neurosurgery 1998;42(3):518–25 [discussion: 525–6].

24. Stummer W, Pichlmeier U, Meinel T, et al. Fluorescence-guided surgery with 5-aminolevulinic acid for resection of malignant glioma: a randomised controlled multicentre phase III trial. Lancet Oncol 2006;7(5):392–401.

25. Stummer W, Novotny A, Stepp H, et al. Fluorescence-guided resection of glioblastoma multiforme by using 5-aminolevulinic acid-induced porphyrins: a prospective study in 52 consecutive patients. J Neurosurg 2000;93(6):1003–13.

26. Stummer W, Suero Molina E. Fluorescence imaging/agents in tumor resection. Neurosurg Clin N Am 2017;28(4):569–83.

27. Stummer W, Reulen HJ, Novotny A, et al. Fluorescence-guided resections of malignant gliomas–an overview. Acta Neurochir Suppl 2003;88:9–12.

28. Stummer W, Rodrigues F, Schucht P, et al. Predicting the "usefulness" of 5-ALA-derived tumor fluorescence for fluorescence-guided resections in pediatric brain tumors: a European survey. Acta Neurochir (Wien) 2014;156(12):2315–24.

29. Stummer W, Stepp H, Wiestler OD, et al. Randomized, prospective double-blinded study comparing 3 different doses of 5-aminolevulinic acid for fluorescence-guided resections of malignant gliomas. Neurosurgery 2017;81(2):230–9.

30. Stummer W, Tonn JC, Goetz C, et al. 5-Aminolevulinic acid-derived tumor fluorescence: the diagnostic accuracy of visible fluorescence qualities as corroborated by spectrometry and histology and postoperative imaging. Neurosurgery 2014;74(3): 310–9 [discussion: 319–20].

31. Widhalm G, Kiesel B, Woehrer A, et al. 5-Aminolevulinic acid induced fluorescence is a powerful intraoperative marker for precise histopathological grading of gliomas with non-significant contrast-enhancement. PLoS One 2013;8(10):e76988.

32. Nishikawa R. Fluorescence illuminates the way. Neuro Oncol 2011;13(8):805.

33. Stockhammer F, Plotkin M, Amthauer H, et al. Correlation of F-18-fluoro-ethyl-tyrosin uptake with vascular and cell density in non-contrast-enhancing gliomas. J Neurooncol 2008;88(2):205–10.

34. Kunz M, Thon N, Eigenbrod S, et al. Hot spots in dynamic (18)FET-PET delineate malignant tumor parts within suspected WHO grade II gliomas. Neuro Oncol 2011;13(3):307–16.

35. Jaber M, Wolfer J, Ewelt C, et al. The value of 5-Aminolevulinic acid in low-grade gliomas and high-grade gliomas lacking glioblastoma imaging features: an analysis based on fluorescence, magnetic resonance imaging, 18F-fluoroethyl tyrosine positron emission tomography, and tumor molecular factors. Neurosurgery 2016;78(3):401–11 [discussion: 411].

36. Suero Molina E, Wolfer J, Ewelt C, et al. Dual-labeling with 5-aminolevulinic acid and fluorescein for fluorescence-guided resection of high-grade gliomas: technical note. J Neurosurg 2018;128(2): 399–405.

37. Suero Molina E, Stummer W. Where and when to cut? Fluorescein guidance for brain stem and spinal cord tumor surgery-technical note. Oper Neurosurg (Hagerstown) 2018;15(3):325–31.

38. Lau D, Hervey-Jumper SL, Chang S, et al. A prospective phase II clinical trial of 5-aminolevulinic acid to assess the correlation of intraoperative fluorescence intensity and degree of histologic cellularity during resection of high-grade gliomas. J Neurosurg 2016;124(5):1300–9.

39. Eberlin LS, Norton I, Orringer D, et al. Ambient mass spectrometry for the intraoperative molecular diagnosis of human brain tumors. Proc Natl Acad Sci U S A 2013;110(5):1611–6.

40. Kut C, Chaichana KL, Xi J, et al. Detection of human brain cancer infiltration ex vivo and in vivo using quantitative optical coherence tomography. Sci Transl Med 2015;7(292):292ra100.

41. Uckermann O, Juratli TA, Galli R, et al. Optical analysis of glioma: Fourier-transform infrared spectroscopy reveals the IDH1 mutation status. Clin Cancer Res 2018;24(11):2530–8.

42. Hollon TC, Orringer DA. Shedding light on IDH1 mutation in gliomas. Clin Cancer Res 2018;24(11): 2467–9.

43. Jermyn M, Mok K, Mercier J, et al. Intraoperative brain cancer detection with Raman spectroscopy in humans. Sci Transl Med 2015;7(274):274ra219.

44. Uckermann O, Galli R, Tamosaityte S, et al. Label-free delineation of brain tumors by coherent anti-Stokes Raman scattering microscopy in an orthotopic mouse model and human glioblastoma. PLoS One 2014;9(9):e107115.

45. Orringer DA, Pandian B, Niknafs YS. Rapid intraoperative histology of unprocessed surgical specimens via fibre-laser-based stimulated Raman scattering microscopy. Nat Biomed Eng 2017;1 [pii:0027].

46. Mizuno A, Kawauchi K, Muraishi S, et al. Near-infrared Fourier transform Raman spectroscopic study of human brain tissues and tumors. J Raman Spectrosc 1994;25:25–9.

47. Koljenovic S, Choo-Smith LP, Bakker Schut TC, et al. Discriminating vital tumor from necrotic tissue in human glioblastoma tissue samples by Raman spectroscopy. Lab Invest 2002;82(10): 1265–77.

48. Kalkanis SN, Kast RE, Rosenblum ML, et al. Raman spectroscopy to distinguish grey matter, necrosis, and glioblastoma multiforme in frozen tissue sections. J Neurooncol 2014;116(3):477–85.

49. Kast R, Auner G, Yurgelevic S, et al. Identification of regions of normal grey matter and white matter from pathologic glioblastoma and necrosis in frozen sections using Raman imaging. J Neurooncol 2015; 125(2):287–95.

50. Kast RE, Auner GW, Rosenblum ML, et al. Raman molecular imaging of brain frozen tissue sections. J Neurooncol 2014;120(1):55–62.

51. Kirsch M, Schackert G, Salzer R, et al. Raman spectroscopic imaging for in vivo detection of cerebral brain metastases. Anal Bioanal Chem 2010;398(4): 1707–13.

52. Jermyn M, Desroches J, Mercier J, et al. Raman spectroscopy detects distant invasive brain cancer cells centimeters beyond MRI capability in humans. Biomed Opt Express 2016;7(12):5129–37.

53. Kaur E, Sahu A, Hole AR, et al. Unique spectral markers discern recurrent Glioblastoma cells from heterogeneous parent population. Sci Rep 2016;6: 26538.

54. Evans CL, Xu X, Kesari S, et al. Chemically-selective imaging of brain structures with CARS microscopy. Opt Express 2007;15(19):12076–87.

55. Camp CH Jr, Lee YJ, Heddleston JM, et al. High-speed coherent Raman fingerprint imaging of biological tissues. Nat Photonics 2014;8: 627–34.

56. Freudiger CW, Min W, Saar BG, et al. Label-free biomedical imaging with high sensitivity by stimulated Raman scattering microscopy. Science 2008; 322(5909):1857–61.

57. Ji M, Lewis S, Camelo-Piragua S, et al. Detection of human brain tumor infiltration with quantitative stimulated Raman scattering microscopy. Sci Transl Med 2015;7(309):309ra163.

58. Hollon TC, Lewis S, Pandian B, et al. Rapid intraoperative diagnosis of pediatric brain tumors using stimulated Raman histology. Cancer Res 2018;7(1): 278–89.

59. Freudiger CW, Yang W, Holtom GR, et al. Stimulated Raman scattering microscopy with a robust fibre laser source. Nat Photonics 2014;8(2):153–9.

Beyond Language
Mapping Cognition and Emotion

Guillaume Herbet, PhD[a,b],*, Sylvie Moritz-Gasser, PhD[a,b]

KEYWORDS

- Intraoperative cognitive mapping • Diffuse low-grade glioma • Emotion • Social cognition
- Semantics • Executive functions • Quality of life • Cognitive recovery

KEY POINTS

- Cognitive mapping during awake surgery has undergone far-reaching changes in recent years.
- Preserving quality of life implies intraoperatively assessing a range of behavioral functions, beyond overt functions such as language or motricity.
- A growing number of medical centers routinely use intraoperative tasks to assess social cognition, emotion, spatial cognition, attention, executive functions, and semantic processing.
- This multifunctional mapping is mandatory to give patients a chance to resume a normal socioprofessional life after surgery.

INTRODUCTION

Intraoperative functional mapping in "awake" surgery is a long-standing surgical technique, widely initiated by Wilder G. Penfield[1] and Georges Ojemann[2,3] in the second half of the twentieth century for epilepsy surgery, then developed by Mitchel Berger[4,5] and Hugues Duffau[6,7] in the context of tumor surgery. The main principles are relatively straightforward: patients are asked to perform a number of behavioral tasks while the neurosurgeon is applying direct electrostimulation on brain structures. If functional disturbances are repeatedly induced during stimulations, the stimulated structure is considered as eloquent for the function under scrutiny; and will then be spared to avoid permanent and debilitating neurologic deficits after surgery. The use of real-time anatomo-functional correlations permitted by direct electrostimulations, especially in glioma surgery, has radically changed the deal. Indeed, it is regularly possible to remove voluminous neoplastic tumors in the so-called eloquent areas (eg, Broca area) without causing any severe and long-lasting neurologic deficits,[8,9] demonstrating that cerebral functions are subserved by complex, distributed, and resilient neural networks, not by discrete and isolated areas.

Although "awake" mapping has historically concerned "overt" functions, such as language or motricity, and has predominantly been applied at the cortical level, this surgical technique has undergone far-reaching changes in recent years. In fact, this rapid development is consubstantial with the greater awareness from neurosurgical physicians that preserving quality of life for patients with a long-survival expectancy (as in low-grade gliomas) cannot not be reduced to the only assessment of functions whose damage leads to overt consequences, such as aphasia or motor defects. As a result, the intraoperative mapping of other important cognitive functions (such as, for example, sociocognitive functions, spatial cognition, and semantic cognition) in both hemispheres has been recently advocated to give the patients the best opportunities of resuming a normal socioprofessional life very promptly after surgery.[10] Moreover, the improvement of subcortical anatomy knowledge, thanks to both the development

Disclosure statement: The authors have nothing to disclose.
[a] Department of Neurosurgery, Montpellier University Medical Center, 80, Avenue Augustin Fliche, Montpellier 34295, France; [b] Institute for Neuroscience of Montpellier, Saint-Eloi Hospital, INSERM U1051, University of Montpellier, 80, Avenue Augustin Fliche, Montpellier 34091, France
* Corresponding author. Gui de Chauliac Hospital, 80, Avenue Augustin Fliche, Montpellier 34295, France.
E-mail address: Guillaume.herbet@gmail.com

of tractography imaging[11,12] and the revival of anatomic dissection,[13,14] and the finding that white matter connections are especially refractory to functional compensation,[15] have prompted "awake" surgery actors to develop cognitive tasks allowing detection of white matter tracts.

In this article, we describe the different behavioral paradigms typically used in "awake" surgery, and how they are selected and modulated to identify and spare the critical pieces of brain-wide cognitive systems.

INTRAOPERATIVE MAPPING AND MONITORING

All the tests presented in this article (except those concerning motor cognition) are administered to the patient intraoperatively by a neuropsychologist/speech therapist on a computer screen, by the means of a slideshow: each slide is presented for 4 seconds (ie, duration of the stimulation effect), and a new slide is announced by a signal tone 500 ms before slide presentation, for the neurosurgeon to know when to apply the stimulation.

It is worth noting that the intraoperative chosen tests are presented a first time to the patient preoperatively.

MOTOR COGNITION

Voluntary movement (ie, the consequence of internal/endogenous activity) engages a set of highly sophisticated neurocognitive processes grouped under the term of motor cognition (ie, intention to act, motor planning, motor initiation, action control). Impairment of motor cognition can lead to a variety of disabling disorders, such as disturbance of bimanual coordination or ideomotor apraxia. A basic way to intraoperatively monitor all aspects of voluntary movement is to ask the patient to perform a dual motor task engaging the upper limb: lower the arm and open the hand, then raise the arm and close the hand (the lower limb may be also concerned or both at the same time). In addition, to control the velocity and the accuracy of the movement during the whole surgery, this task enables mapping under stimulation crucial areas for motor cognition.[16] Depending on the structures being stimulated, several neuropsychological impairments can be observed: for example, stimulation of the supplementary motor area can lead to motor initiation disturbances. Other motor tasks also can be performed to map more specific motor abilities. Regularly, we ask the patients to make coordinated movements with both hands,[17,18] an ability especially crucial for certain professions (eg, manual work, musician). It is also important

to ask the patient to perform more complex movements to assess fine-grained motor abilities, such as drumming, or to perform reflexive praxis (eg, imitation of meaningless movements) to evaluate movement planning.

The consistent use of these behavioral tasks during intraoperative electrostimulation has allowed us to gain considerable insight into the network mediating (voluntary) motor control (the negative motor network). Data from stimulation mapping has indeed permitted determination of the spatial topography, both at the cortical and subcortical levels, of this apparently widely distributed neural system. Briefly, the network is formed by the supplementary motor area and the lateral premotor cortex, these regions being interconnected via the frontal aslant tract and with the head of the caudate via the fronto-striatal tract. Some of these projection fibers run toward the anterior arm of the internal capsule. A subnetwork interconnects the precentral with the retrocentral gyri via U-fibers passing deep in the central region. Disruption of the negative motor network has important consequences on movement control and initiation (including speech-related motor processes).

BASIC VISUAL PROCESSES

Patients with a large visual field defect, such as lateral homonymous hemianopia (HLH), have generally a poor functional outcome. In many countries, driving is formally prohibited and many activities, such as reading, become arduous. To map visual connectivity and avoid the occurrence of long-term postoperative visual field defects, we use a simple protocol allowing assessment of visual fields during surgery.[19] Specifically, with the vision being fixed on a red cross at the center of the computer screen, patients are asked to name successively 2 pictures displayed in the 2 opposite quadrants, keeping in mind that it is absolutely crucial to preserve the inferior quadrant, the superior one being compensable in daily life. The position of the pictures is determined by the laterality of the lesion. Although direct electrical stimulation of visual pathways, especially the optic radiations, generally evokes a range a phenomena subjectively described by the patient (either "inhibitory phenomena," such as blurred vision or impression of shadow, or "excitatory phenomena," such as phosphenes), the described task allows a more objective confirmation of the transitory visual disturbance induced (ie, the patient cannot see the picture presented in the inferior quadrant contralateral to the lesion). Some indicators are also important to take into consideration during the assessment of visual fields, notably the amplitude of visual saccades or the possible increase of naming response time in the visual field under scrutiny. During the resection, it is moreover mandatory to regularly check manually the visual field with basic neurologic tests.

VISUAL COGNITION

The inferolateral occipito-temporal pathway is reputed to broadcast critical information in the service of object recognition.[20] Damage to this neural system may lead to visual agnosia: a disabling inability of visually recognizing objects. A simple way to map these high-order visual processes during awake surgery is to use a picture-naming task. If a disturbance of object recognition is induced during electrostimulation, the patient generally commits a non–semantically related "visual" paraphasia (eg, "drum" for "stool").

Our group has previously shown that axonal stimulation of the inferior longitudinal fasciculus (ILF), which interconnects the occipital and temporo-occipital areas with the lateral and medial portions of the temporal pole, leads to contralateral visual hemiagnosia,[20,21] demonstrating the vital role of this white matter connectivity in conveying high-level visual information. It is worth mentioning that visual agnosia is generally generated in the right hemisphere, not in the left hemisphere where stimulation or lesion-induced damage of the ILF rather leads to alexia[22] or lexical retrieval difficulties.[23,24] Note that the bilateral disruption of the ILF can lead to other forms of visual agnosia, in particular prosopagnosia,[25] an inability to recognize familiar faces. This is consistent with recent evidence that this contingent of white matter fibers is specifically atrophied in patients with congenital prosopagnosia.[26,27]

VISUOSPATIAL COGNITION

Unilateral spatial neglect is a debilitating neurologic condition characterized by a failure to explore and allocate attention in the space contralateral to the damaged hemisphere. It may occur after lesion of many cortical brain territories, especially in the right hemisphere.[28] This cognitive impairment has a major impact on quality of life by depriving the patient to resume a normal social and professional life.

A classic test to evaluate spatial neglect is the line bisection task. For surgery, we have adapted this task in a touch-screen environment. The patient is asked to separate a line into 2 identical segments (ie, find the true center of the line). The length of the line is usually 18 cm. If, during the time of stimulation, a significant rightward deviation (for a tumor in the right hemisphere) is induced (typically 7 mm or slightly more if the patient presents with a behavioral variability), the brain area under scrutiny is considered as eloquent for visuospatial cognition.[29]

The line bisection task is useful to map the posterior parietal cortex, including the inferior and superior parietal lobules, but also to a lesser extent the posterior temporal cortex.[30–32] Most importantly, it enables identification of the dorsal white matter connectivity, especially the layer II of the superior longitudinal fasciculus (SLF) in the right hemisphere. This white matter tract, by interconnecting the superior and inferior parietal lobules (and the cortex within the intraparietal sulcus) with the posterior middle frontal gyrus[33,34] is thought to maintain information exchange between the ventral and the dorsal attention system,[35] and is strongly associated with spatial neglect in case of neurologic insult.[36] Using the same behavioral paradigm, a recent electrostimulation study has shown that the right inferior fronto-occipital fasciculus (IFOF), a brain-wide white matter tract providing connections between the occipital, parietal, and temporal lobes and the prefrontal cortex also may play a role in spatial cognition,[37] as previously hypothesized but not clearly behaviorally evidenced. This is consistent with the emerging view that the IFOF may support a multilayered organization. More specifically, the IFOF may be organized in 2[13,38] or even more streams[39] (ie, 5) having projections to cortical structures known to be involved in spatial cognition, such as the posterior dorsolateral prefrontal cortex, the superior parietal lobule, the angular gyrus, and the posterior part of the temporal gyrus. Thus, it is possible that 1 or maybe more of the IFOF layers are specifically devoted to some aspects of spatial cognition/attention, especially layers connecting the ventrolateral prefrontal (ie, IFOF-III[39]) or the posterior dorsolateral prefrontal cortex (ie, deep layer[13] or IFOF-IV[39]) to the posterior parietal cortex (ie, superior parietal lobule and angular gyrus).

In brief, the use of a simple line bisection task allows mapping and preserving of critical structures for spatial attention. A recent study performed by our group has shown that, although approximately half of the patients with a right tumor experienced a transitory neglect in the immediate postoperative phase, none of them presented a persistent spatial neglect, demonstrating greatly the effectiveness of this intraoperative mapping.

DUAL-TASKING AND MULTITASKING

Numerous activities in daily life necessitate processing different matters at the same time. This crucial multitasking ability requires maintaining in working memory several task goals to be performed and concurrently allocating attention among them. During surgery, this higher capacity can be assessed by asking the patient to perform simultaneously a regular movement of the upper limb and a naming task or a semantic association task. A multitasking disturbance is observed when the patient is no longer able to perform both tasks at the same time, although the realization of each task separately remains possible. This impairment, to a lesser extent, may be manifested in a temporary desynchronization/lack of coordination between both tasks.

SOCIAL COGNITION AND EMOTION

Human beings are especially talented in understanding and predicting others' behavior. This complex ability, commonly referred to as "mentalizing" or "Theory of Mind," is one of the main foundations on which social cognition is built[40] and is unsurprisingly disrupted in a wide range of neuropsychiatric conditions, especially those in which social communication is highly problematic, such as autism spectrum disorders and schizophrenia. Mentalizing is not a unitary process, but rather encompasses a variety of more basic, and for some nonspecific, subprocesses, such as emotion processing, inferential reasoning, understanding of causality, and self/other distinction.[41] Patients with social cognition disorders have difficulties understanding their social environment, leading to abnormal behaviors (ie, acquired sociopathy) and lack of social flexibility.

To avoid long-term and debilitating postoperative social cognition impairments, we use during awake surgery an adapted version of a well-tried mentalizing task (ie, The Read the Mind in the Eyes Task[42]). The original version of this behavioral task consists of the presentation of 36 photographs depicting the eye region of human faces. For each of them, 4 affective states are suggested and participants are asked to select the one that best describes what the person on the photograph is currently feeling or thinking. This behavioral task enables tapping of the lower, prereflective, and automatic (as opposed to high-level, reflective, inferential) aspect of mentalizing. We have indeed shown that patients with a resection of the pars opercularis of the right inferior frontal gyrus did not completely recover after surgery,[43,44] justifying clinically the use of a new intraoperative task

(Fig. 1A). Consistent with previous literature using face-based mentalizing tasks,[45] crucial cortical epicenters are regularly identified, with, however, some degree of interindividual variability, in the posterior inferior frontal gyrus, the dorsolateral prefrontal cortex, and the posterior superior temporal gyrus.[46] More importantly, critical sites are also pinpointed along the inferior IFOF, and within the white matter fibers supplying the dorsolateral prefrontal cortex,[46] suggesting that functional integrity of both the direct ventral connectivity and the dorsal connectivity via the SLF are required for accurately inferring complex mental states from human faces.

LANGUAGE AND SEMANTICS

To map language processes, the use of a naming task remains the gold standard. This task, which is easy to implement during surgery and is especially adapted to patient positioning constraints, is very sensitive to all levels of language and speech processing. During electrostimulation, different kinds of impairments may be observed: speech arrest, anarthria (disturbance of motor programming), anomia (disturbance of lexical retrieval: the patient is unable to name the object), phonological paraphasia (disturbance of phonological encoding: production of a word with phonological deviations, eg, phelephant for elephant), semantic paraphasia (disturbance of semantic processing, production of a word semantically related to the target word, eg, cow for horse), disfluencies or stuttering (disturbance of speech initiation), or perseveration (disturbance of inhibitory control mechanisms, repetition of a prior word in front of a new picture[47]). Beyond classic language-related cortical areas, the naming task enables mapping of the main associative connectivities (ie, the arcuate fasciculus for phonological processes, the anterior lateral SLF for articulatory processes, the IFOF for semantic control processes [see later in this article], and the ILF for lexical retrieval[23,24]) and certain intralobar tracts, such as the frontal aslant tract (speech initiation and control).[48]

To intraoperatively assess the nonverbal semantic system (the naming task enables only assessment of verbal semantics), we also routinely use a semantic association task (ie, the Pyramids and Palm Trees Test[49]). This task consists of 52 black and white drawn pictures; for each target picture, 2 new pictures are proposed and the patient is asked to match one or both with the target one according to a semantic link, by pointing it out. We have previously shown that this task is useful to map and preserve the direct ventral connectivity, especially the IFOF in the left hemisphere,[50]

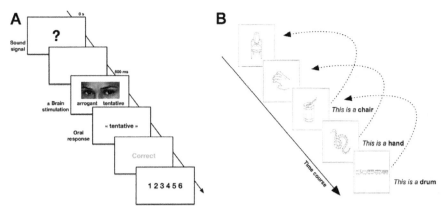

Fig. 1. Examples of intraoperative tasks. (*A*) Mentalizing task (assessment of social cognition). (*B*) n-back task (assessment of working memory).

but also in the right hemisphere.[51] This is consistent with the fact that cortical epicenters for nonverbal semantics are mainly distributed in the dorsolateral prefrontal cortex,[52] a cortical structure that is densely interconnected by the IFOF.

When the tumor concerns the left occipitotemporal cortex, especially the visual word-forming area and its underlying white matter connectivity (especially the posterior part of the left ILF and posterior aspect of the arcuate fasciculus), it is necessary to map the different subprocesses involved in reading aloud. To this end, we typically use a reading task in which the patient is asked to read aloud different word categories; that is, regular and irregular words, and pseudo-words.[22] Finally, to map brain areas involved in the motor implementation of automatic speech production, we routinely use a counting task consisting of counting aloud from 1 to 10 in loop.

On the basis of electrostimulation mapping findings, our group has recently proposed a dynamic dual-stream anatomofunctional model for language processing[53] with a ventral stream involved in mapping visual information to meaning (semantics) and a dorsal stream dedicated to mapping visual information to articulation through visuo-phonological conversion. Compared with other neurocognitive or computational models,[54] this model has the great advantage of incorporating anatomic constraints, especially white matter connectivity information.

CONSCIOUS INFORMATION PROCESSING

Based on patients' behavior, electrostimulation can be used to identify critical cerebral structures involved in the maintenance of conscious information processing. For example, our group has shown in a single patient that stimulation of the white matter emanating from the dorsal posterior

cingulate cortex induces a breakdown in conscious experience characterized by a transient behavioral unresponsiveness with loss of external connectedness (retrospectively, the patient described himself as in a dream, outside the operating room[55,56]), a modified state of consciousness that is very similar to what it is observed in rapid eye movement sleep. This finding was recently replicated in 3 other patients.[56] Taken as a whole, these observations suggest that functional integrity of the posterior cingulate connectivity is absolutely necessary to maintain consciousness of the external environment.

INDIVIDUALIZED TASKS

Some patients have a strong expertise in some cognitive domains due to their occupation or their hobbies (numerical cognition in a mathematician expert, working memory in a management assistant, some are bilingual or trilingual). In such cases, specific tasks can be built and implemented to ensure that some important aspects of cognitive functioning are not impaired and that the patient will recover promptly a normal professional life after surgery. For example, an n-back task (**Fig. 1**B), which consists of naming the picture viewed n trials before, can be used to assess short-term and working memory: the capacity to maintain and manipulate information to achieve a particular goal. This kind of behavioral paradigm is useful to identify and spare the frontal-parietal network mediated by the SLF. Alternatively, some groups conduct the assessment of working memory with a classic span task.[57]

Simple numerical cognition tasks can be used to assess basic mathematical operations. This is done by asking the patient to resolve simple operations (such as 6 + 5; 15 − 6) on auditory-verbal or visual inputs. This is useful to map the posterior parietal cortex, especially in the left hemisphere.

Finally, in rare cases of professional musicians, music production tasks can be performed to sustain the patient's abilities.[58]

FUTURE DEVELOPMENTS FOR THE INTRAOPERATIVE MAPPING OF COGNITIVE FUNCTIONS

An issue frequently raised by actors of "awake" surgery relates to the use of alternative behavioral tasks for the intraoperative mapping and monitoring, such as more fine-grained linguistic or memory tasks[57,59,60] or executive function tasks.[61] However, the choice of implementing new behavior paradigms in standard practice certainly deserves a few considerations:

- First, the cognitive paradigms previously described appear to be sufficient to map both the cortical structures and the main white matter connectivities that are refractory to functional compensation.[15]
- Second, the intraoperative tasks must be necessarily simple and easily workable given the constraints related to the electrostimulation procedure (stimulation duration: 4 seconds maximum), the clinical context (intraoperative mapping cannot be too long), and the patient's position in the operating theater. For example, highly integrated functions are widely distributed at the brain level and require coordination of activity of multiple networks.[62] These functions, such as cognitive flexibility, are therefore likely to be difficult to map during "awake" surgery.
- Third, the best onco-functional balance must be found: the first goal toward the surgery is to optimize the extent of resection while preserving quality of life. Adding too many tasks might eventually affect the achievement of surgery.
- Fourth, before adding new intraoperative tasks, longitudinal studies (before and a few months after surgery) are needed to assess the extent to which patients recover on a wide range of cognitive and socio-affective functions. If patients do not recover sufficiently, despite intensive and individualized postoperative rehabilitation, and are impeded in their daily life functioning, there is some rationale in developing new well-controlled and easily "standardizable" tasks. Clearly, only a handful of research groups has provided this kind of very important study.[43,63–65]
- Finally, the pathophysiological mechanisms of the lack of recovery after surgery need to be better understood. Indeed, cognitive disorders after surgery could be equally explained by other factors than the surgical procedure itself, such as the degree of infiltration of white matter connectivity,[44,57,66] the growth rate of the tumor, the preoperative functional status, the interindividual variability in the neuroplasticity potential,[67] the socio-educational level, and probably the patient's personality.

SUMMARY

In this review, we described the main behavioral paradigms typically used in the operating theater to map and spare critical brain structures devoted to important aspects of cognitive functioning, in both the left and right hemispheres. As a final note, we wish to make clear that cognitive brain mapping is just a particular step in the clinical management and is not sufficient by itself to guarantee the patients a complete functional recovery. In fact, it is hugely important that patients benefit from comprehensive neuropsychological investigations both before and just after surgery to assess to what extent functions are eventually impaired. The comparison between the preoperative and the postoperative cognitive status allows tailoring of personalized cognitive rehabilitation, which considerably increases the probability of complete recovery. Controlled studies demonstrating the merits of this approach are still, however, lacking, but could provide better guidance for postoperative management.

REFERENCES

1. Penfield W, Boldrey E. Somatic motor and sensory representation in the cerebral cortex of man as studied by electrical stimulation. Brain 1937;60(4): 389–443.
2. Ojemann GA. Individual variability in cortical localization of language. J Neurosurg 1979;50(2):164–9.
3. Ojemann GA, Whitaker HA. Language localization and variability. Brain Lang 1978;6(2):239–60.
4. Berger MS, Ojemann GA, Lettich E. Neurophysiological monitoring during astrocytoma surgery. Neurosurg Clin N Am 1990;1(1):65–80.
5. Berger MS, Ojemann GA. Intraoperative brain mapping techniques in neuro-oncology. Stereotact Funct Neurosurg 1992;58(1–4):153–61.
6. Duffau H, Capelle L, Sichez N, et al. Intraoperative mapping of the subcortical language pathways using direct stimulations: an anatomo-functional study. Brain 2002;125(1):199–214.
7. Duffau H. Lessons from brain mapping in surgery for low-grade glioma: insights into associations between tumour and brain plasticity. Lancet Neurol 2005;4(8):476–86.

8. Plaza M, Gatignol P, Leroy M, et al. Speaking without Broca's area after tumor resection. Neurocase 2009; 15(4):294–310.

9. Sarubbo S, Le Bars E, Moritz-Gasser S, et al. Complete recovery after surgical resection of left Wernicke's area in awake patient: a brain stimulation and functional MRI study. Neurosurg Rev 2012; 35(2):287–92.

10. Vilasboas T, Herbet G, Duffau H. Challenging the myth of right "non-dominant" hemisphere: lessons from cortico-subcortical stimulation mapping in awake surgery and surgical implications. World Neurosurg 2017;103:449–56.

11. Basser PJ, Pajevic S, Pierpaoli C, et al. In vivo fiber tractography using DT-MRI data. Magn Reson Med 2000;44(4):625–32.

12. Catani M, Howard RJ, Pajevic S, et al. Virtual in vivo interactive dissection of white matter fasciculi in the human brain. Neuroimage 2002;17(1):77–94.

13. Sarubbo S, De Benedictis A, Maldonado IL, et al. Frontal terminations for the inferior fronto-occipital fascicle: anatomical dissection, DTI study and functional considerations on a multi-component bundle. Brain Struct Funct 2013;218(1):21–37.

14. Maldonado IL, Champfleur NM, Velut S, et al. Evidence of a middle longitudinal fasciculus in the human brain from fiber dissection. J Anat 2013; 223(1):38–45.

15. Herbet G, Maheu M, Costi E, et al. Mapping neuroplastic potential in brain-damaged patients. Brain 2016;139(3):829–44.

16. Schucht P, Moritz-Gasser S, Herbet G, et al. Subcortical electrostimulation to identify network subserving motor control. Hum Brain Mapp 2013;34(11): 3023–30.

17. Rech F, Herbet G, Moritz-Gasser S, et al. Somatotopic organization of the white matter tracts underpinning motor control in humans: an electrical stimulation study. Brain Struct Funct 2016;221(7): 3743–53.

18. Rech F, Herbet G, Moritz-Gasser S, et al. Disruption of bimanual movement by unilateral subcortical electrostimulation. Hum Brain Mapp 2014;35(7): 3439–45.

19. Gras-Combe G, Moritz-Gasser S, Herbet G, et al. Intraoperative subcortical electrical mapping of optic radiations in awake surgery for glioma involving visual pathways. J Neurosurg 2012;117(3):466–73.

20. Mandonnet E, Gatignol P, Duffau H. Evidence for an occipito-temporal tract underlying visual recognition in picture naming. Clin Neurol Neurosurg 2009; 111(7):601–5.

21. Coello AF, Duvaux S, De Benedictis A, et al. Involvement of the right inferior longitudinal fascicle in visual hemiagnosia: a brain stimulation mapping study: case report. J Neurosurg 2013; 118(1):202–5.

22. Zemmoura I, Blanchard E, Raynal P-I, et al. How Klingler's dissection permits exploration of brain structural connectivity? An electron microscopy study of human white matter. Brain Struct Funct 2016;221(5):2477–86.

23. Herbet G, Moritz-Gasser S, Lemaitre A-L, et al. Functional compensation of the left inferior longitudinal fasciculus for picture naming. Cogn Neuropsychol 2018;1–18. https://doi.org/10.1080/02643294. 2018.1477749.

24. Herbet G, Moritz-Gasser S, Boiseau M, et al. Converging evidence for a cortico-subcortical network mediating lexical retrieval. Brain 2016; 139(11):3007–21.

25. Corrivetti F, Herbet G, Moritz-Gasser S, et al. Prosopagnosia induced by a left anterior temporal lobectomy following a right temporo-occipital resection in a multicentric diffuse low-grade glioma. World Neurosurg 2017;97:756.e1–5.

26. Thomas C, Avidan G, Humphreys K, et al. Reduced structural connectivity in ventral visual cortex in congenital prosopagnosia. Nat Neurosci 2009; 12(1):29–31.

27. Grossi D, Soricelli A, Ponari M, et al. Structural connectivity in a single case of progressive prosopagnosia: the role of the right inferior longitudinal fasciculus. Cortex 2014;56:111–20.

28. Molenberghs P, Cunnington R, Mattingley JB. Brain regions with mirror properties: a meta-analysis of 125 human fMRI studies. Neurosci Biobehav Rev 2012;36(1):341–9.

29. Bartolomeo P, de Schotten MT, Duffau H. Mapping of visuospatial functions during brain surgery: a new tool to prevent unilateral spatial neglect. Neurosurgery 2007;61(6):E1340.

30. Roux F-E, Dufor O, Lauwers-Cances V, et al. Electrostimulation mapping of spatial neglect. Neurosurgery 2011;69(6):1218–31.

31. Vallar G, Bello L, Bricolo E, et al. Cerebral correlates of visuospatial neglect: a direct cerebral stimulation study. Hum Brain Mapp 2014;35(4):1334–50.

32. Thiebaut de Schotten M, Urbanski M, Duffau H, et al. Direct evidence for a parietal-frontal pathway subserving spatial awareness in humans. Science 2005;309(5744):2226–8.

33. Makris N, Kennedy DN, McInerney S, et al. Segmentation of subcomponents within the superior longitudinal fascicle in humans: a quantitative, in vivo, DT-MRI study. Cereb Cortex 2004;15(6):854–69.

34. Schmahmann JD, Pandya DN, Wang R, et al. Association fibre pathways of the brain: parallel observations from diffusion spectrum imaging and autoradiography. Brain 2007;130(3):630–53.

35. Bartolomeo P, De Schotten MT, Chica AB. Brain networks of visuospatial attention and their disruption in visual neglect. Front Hum Neurosci 2012;6:110.

36. Thiebaut de Schotten M, Tomaiuolo F, Aiello M, et al. Damage to white matter pathways in subacute and chronic spatial neglect: a group study and 2 single-case studies with complete virtual "in vivo" tractography dissection. Cereb Cortex 2012;24(3):691–706.

37. Herbet G, Yordanova YN, Duffau H. Left spatial neglect evoked by electrostimulation of the right inferior fronto-occipital fasciculus. Brain Topogr 2017;30(6):747–56.

38. Hau J, Sarubbo S, Perchey G, et al. Cortical terminations of the inferior fronto-occipital and uncinate fasciculi: anatomical stem-based virtual dissection. Front Neuroanat 2016;10:58.

39. Wu Y, Sun D, Wang Y, et al. Subcomponents and connectivity of the inferior fronto-occipital fasciculus revealed by diffusion spectrum imaging fiber tracking. Front Neuroanat 2016;10:88.

40. Lieberman MD. Social cognitive neuroscience: a review of core processes. Annu Rev Psychol 2007;58:259–89.

41. Schaafsma SM, Pfaff DW, Spunt RP, et al. Deconstructing and reconstructing theory of mind. Trends Cogn Sci 2015;19(2):65–72.

42. Baron-Cohen S, Wheelwright S, Hill J, et al. The "Reading the Mind in the Eyes" Test revised version: a study with normal adults, and adults with Asperger syndrome or high-functioning autism. J Child Psychol Psychiatry 2001;42(2):241–51.

43. Herbet G, Lafargue G, Bonnetblanc F, et al. Is the right frontal cortex really crucial in the mentalizing network? A longitudinal study in patients with a slow-growing lesion. Cortex 2013;49(10):2711–27.

44. Herbet G, Lafargue G, Bonnetblanc F, et al. Inferring a dual-stream model of mentalizing from associative white matter fibres disconnection. Brain 2014;137(3):944–59.

45. Schurz M, Radua J, Aichhorn M, et al. Fractionating theory of mind: a meta-analysis of functional brain imaging studies. Neurosci Biobehav Rev 2014;42:9.

46. Yordanova YN, Duffau H, Herbet G. Neural pathways subserving face-based mentalizing. Brain Struct Funct 2017;222(7):3087–105.

47. Duffau H, Gatignol P, Mandonnet E, et al. New insights into the anatomo-functional connectivity of the semantic system: a study using cortico-subcortical electrostimulations. Brain 2005;128(4):797–810.

48. Kinoshita M, de Champfleur NM, Deverdun J, et al. Role of fronto-striatal tract and frontal aslant tract in movement and speech: an axonal mapping study. Brain Struct Funct 2015;220(6):3399–412.

49. Howard D, Patterson KE. The pyramids and palm trees test: a test of semantic access from words and pictures. Bury St Edmunds: Thames Valley Test Company; 1992.

50. Moritz-Gasser S, Herbet G, Duffau H. Mapping the connectivity underlying multimodal (verbal and non-verbal) semantic processing: a brain electrostimulation study. Neuropsychologia 2013;51(10):1814–22.

51. Herbet G, Moritz-Gasser S, Duffau H. Direct evidence for the contributive role of the right inferior fronto-occipital fasciculus in non-verbal semantic cognition. Brain Struct Funct 2017;222(4):1597–610.

52. Herbet G, Moritz-Gasser S, Duffau H. Electrical stimulation of the dorsolateral prefrontal cortex impairs semantic cognition. Neurology 2018;90(12):e1077–84.

53. Duffau H, Herbet G, Moritz-Gasser S. Toward a pluri-component, multimodal, and dynamic organization of the ventral semantic stream in humans: lessons from stimulation mapping in awake patients. Front Syst Neurosci 2013;7:44.

54. Hickok G, Poeppel D. Dorsal and ventral streams: a framework for understanding aspects of the functional anatomy of language. Cognition 2004;92(1):67–99.

55. Herbet G, Lafargue G, De Champfleur NM, et al. Disrupting posterior cingulate connectivity disconnects consciousness from the external environment. Neuropsychologia 2014;56:239–44.

56. Herbet G, Lafargue G, Duffau H. The dorsal cingulate cortex as a critical gateway in the network supporting conscious awareness. Brain 2015;139(4):e23.

57. Papagno C, Comi A, Riva M, et al. Mapping the brain network of the phonological loop. Hum Brain Mapp 2017;38(6):3011–24.

58. Leonard MK, Desai M, Hungate D, et al. Direct cortical stimulation of inferior frontal cortex disrupts both speech and music production in highly trained musicians. Cogn Neuropsychol 2018;1–9. https://doi.org/10.1080/02643294.2018.1472559.

59. Rofes A, Miceli G. Language mapping with verbs and sentences in awake surgery: a review. Neuropsychol Rev 2014;24(2):185–99.

60. Orena EF, Caldiroli D, Acerbi F, et al. Investigating the functional neuroanatomy of concrete and abstract word processing through direct electric stimulation (DES) during awake surgery. Cogn Neuropsychol 2018;1–11. https://doi.org/10.1080/02643294.2018.1477748.

61. Mandonnet E, Cerliani L, Siuda-Krzywicka K, et al. A network-level approach of cognitive flexibility impairment after surgery of a right temporo-parietal glioma. Neurochirurgie 2017;63(4):308–13.

62. Cocchi L, Zalesky A, Fornito A, et al. Dynamic cooperation and competition between brain systems during cognitive control. Trends Cogn Sci 2013;17(10):493–501.

63. Charras P, Herbet G, Deverdun J, et al. Functional reorganization of the attentional networks in low-grade glioma patients: a longitudinal study. Cortex 2015;63:27–41.

64. Nakajima R, Kinoshita M, Miyashita K, et al. Damage of the right dorsal superior longitudinal fascicle by awake surgery for glioma causes

persistent visuospatial dysfunction. Sci Rep 2017; 7(1):17158.

65. Wilson SM, Lam D, Babiak MC, et al. Transient aphasias after left hemisphere resective surgery. J Neurosurg 2015;123(3):581–93.

66. Nakajima R, Yordanova YN, Duffau H, et al. Neuropsychological evidence for the crucial role of the right arcuate fasciculus in the face-based mentalizing network: a disconnection analysis. Neuropsychologia 2018;115:179–87.

67. Duffau H. A two-level model of interindividual anatomo-functional variability of the brain and its implications for neurosurgery. Cortex 2017;86: 303–13.

Evidence for Improving Outcome Through Extent of Resection

Shawn L. Hervey-Jumper, MD[a],*, Mitchel S. Berger, MD[b]

KEYWORDS

• Extent of resection • Volume of residual • Low-grade glioma • Astrocytoma • Oligodendroglioma

KEY POINTS

• Greater extent of tumor resection influences overall and malignant progression-free survival in patients with World Health Organization 2 gliomas.
• The significance of Extent of Resection (EOR) across varying molecular glioma subtype remains unknown.
• Although maximal resection influences survival, the presence of functional language and motor deficits negatively impacts overall survival; therefore, EOR must be balanced against functional outcomes.

AN EVIDENCE-BASED APPROACH TO MAXIMAL SAFE RESECTION

There has been great interest in the significance of maximal resection for gliomas for more than 30 years. Gliomas are a major cause of morbidity and mortality in the United States,[1] and low-grade gliomas (World Health Organization [WHO] grades II astrocytoma and oligodendrogliomas) have proven difficult to treat due to their propensity to infiltrate deep into surrounding parenchyma. An increasing body of evidence suggests that greater extent of resection and lower volume of tumor residual extends both overall (OS) and progression-free survival (PFS). Extent of tumor resection in addition to younger patient age, tumor histology (oligodendroglioma vs astrocytoma), patient functional status, and molecular subclassification (1p19q codeletion, isocitrate dehydrogenase [IDH] 1 or 2 mutation status) are predictive of outcome.[2–7] Cytoreduction through maximal resection plays a central role in the management of gliomas. In addition, there is recent evidence that supercomplete resection, when possible, offers an additional survival benefit[8] (see Hugues Duffau's article, "Higher Order Surgical Questions for Diffuse Low-Grade Gliomas: Supramaximal Resection, Neuroplasticity and Screening," in this issue). However, gross total or supercomplete resection can be difficult to achieve in many cases due to glioma infiltration into cortical and subcortical regions significant for language, motor, and neurocognitive function.

Numerous published studies have increased the understanding of the value of surgery for low-grade gliomas (**Table 1**). Since 1990, 30 studies have focused on the worth of extent of resection to improve OS and PFS in patients with low-grade astrocytomas and oligodendrogliomas (see **Table 1**).[3–6,9–30] Early reports focused on

Disclosure Statement: Dr Hervey-Jumper and Berger are supported by NCI SPORE grant number 5P50CA097257-15.
[a] Department of Neurological Surgery, University of California San Francisco, 513 Parnassus Avenue, Health Sciences East Suite 814, San Francisco, CA 94143-0112, USA; [b] Department of Neurological Surgery, University of California San Francisco, 505 Parnassus Avenue, M779, San Francisco, CA 94143-0112, USA
* Corresponding author.
E-mail address: Shawn.Hervey-Jumper@ucsf.edu

Neurosurg Clin N Am 30 (2019) 85–93
https://doi.org/10.1016/j.nec.2018.08.005
1042-3680/19/© 2018 Elsevier Inc. All rights reserved.

Table 1
Summary of literature including extent of resection in low-grade (World Health Organization grade 2) glioma

OS	Nonvolumetric Studies	No. of Patients	Volumetric Studies	No. of Patients
Benefit	North et al,[17] 1990	77	van Veelen et al,[26] 1998	75
	Philippon et al,[19] 1993	179	Claus et al,[10] 2005	156
	Rajan et al,[20] 1994	82	Smith et al,[24] 2008	216
	Leighton et al,[16] 1997	167	Sanai & Berger,[21] 2008	104
	Nakamura et al.,[4] 2000	88	Incekara et al,[12] 2016	128
	Yeh et al,[28] 2005	93	Hollon et al,[11] 2016	109
	McGirt et al.,[52] 2009	170	Snyder et al,[25] 2014	93
	Ahmadi et al.,[51] 2009	130	Wijnenga et al,[30] 2018	228
	Chaichana et al,[66] 2013	191	Patel et al,[29] 2018	74
	Jakola et al,[32] 2012	153		
	Lote et al,[3] 1997	379		
	Nicolato et al,[5] 1995	76		
	Scerrati et al,[6] 1996	131		
	Ito et al,[13] 1994	89		
	Karim et al,[15] 1996	311		
	Peraud et al,[18] 1998	75		
	Shaw et al,[22] 2002	203		
	Shibamoto et al,[23] 1993	178		
No Benefit	Whitton & Bloom,[27] 1990	88	None to date	
	Bauman et al,[9] 1999	401		
	Johannesen et al,[14] 2003	993		

estimates of extent of resection based on neurosurgery and radiology reports, whereas more recent data use detailed volumetric assessments. The introduction of the revised WHO 2016 classification of gliomas requires a reassessment of the survival of grade 2 glioma patients along molecular definitions. Taken together, the reported median OS in *IDH mutant* WHO 2 astrocytoma is in the 9- to 10-year range, and in *IDH* mutant 1p/19q codeleted oligodendrogliomas may be more than 14 years.[31] The added survival when considering all WHO 2 gliomas (regardless of molecular subgroup) with gross total resection (GTR) ranges between 61.1 and 90 months. However, current reports are limited by short follow-up periods.

Maximal upfront resection of WHO 2 gliomas became firmly established following publication of a large population-based study of Norwegian patients, which offered analysis of 153 glioma patients treated in 2 hospitals serving adjacent geographic regions.[32] The approach to the care of gliomas in individualized patients was dependent on residential address, which consistently varied between the 2 hospitals included in the study. The neuro-oncology team from hospital "A" favored biopsy followed by watchful waiting, whereas hospital "B" offered upfront maximal safe resection at the time of diagnosis. Patients were matched for clinical demographics, such as patient age, baseline health status, and

baseline glioma volumes. Median survival in this study was 5.9 years for patients receiving biopsy only, whereas the group receiving early resection did not reach median survival by the end of the study period, suggesting a survival benefit for those treated with early surgery. Furthermore, 5-year survival was 60% for biopsy patients and 74% for those receiving early surgery.[32] The survival benefit for early resection is thought to be due to identifying gliomas of smaller size with a greater likelihood of GTR.[33,34] Therefore, surgical resection is now considered for incidentally identified presumed low-grade gliomas (see Hugues Duffau's article, "Higher Order Surgical Questions for Diffuse Low-Grade Gliomas: Supramaximal Resection, Neuroplasticity and Screening," in this issue). Maximal resection of the T2 or fluid-attenuated inversion recovery (FLAIR) signal extent of infiltrating glioma, as detected on preoperative MRI, is thought to positively influence the natural history of low-grade gliomas. In addition, removal of a margin around the glioma (considered supratotal resection) might improve outcome even further when compared with GTR.[8]

Malignant transformation of low-grade gliomas ranges from 4 to 29 months, and roughly 45% of patients with diffuse low-grade WHO grade 2 glioma will undergo transformation to anaplastic (WHO grade 3) glioma within 5 years.[24,25,35–37] The question has always remained as to whether an extent of resection or volume of residual threshold can be determined. When considering surgical interventions, this question is particularly important, given the fact that many WHO 2 gliomas occur within areas of presumed eloquence. Many times patients will present initially with diffuse nonfocal tumors, so the decision must be made upfront whether to consider maximal resection versus biopsy, and to what extent (**Fig. 1**). Smith and colleagues[24] analyzed 216 patients with hemispheric low-grade gliomas. After adjusting for age, performance status, and tumor location, extent of resection remained a significant predictor of OS and malignant progression-free survival (MPFS); however, only a trend toward longer progression-free survival was observed. Patients with at least 90% extent of resection experienced 5- and 8-year OS, progression-free, and MPFS rates of 97% and 91%, 75% and 43%, and 93% and 76%, respectively. Conversely, patients receiving less than 90% extent of resection had 5- and 8-year OS, PFS, and MPFS rates of 76% and 60%, 40% and 21%, and 72% and 48%, respectively. Furthermore, complete removal of all FLAIR abnormality resulted in 98% 5- and 8-year OS with 79% of patients without malignant transformation.[24] Smith and colleagues[24] in their analysis used extent of resection as a categorical, not continuous variable. However, they were able to illustrate extent of resection as a significant predictor of OS even when their cohort of patients was limited to only individuals with greater than 80% extent of resection.[24]

Claus and colleagues[10] in a follow-up study reported that patients who underwent incomplete resection of WHO 2 gliomas were at 4.9 times the risk of death relative to patients with GTR. Similar to Smith and colleagues,[10,24] they found a statistical EOR cutoff, again using EOR as a categorical variable, at 90%. However, the survival benefit continued down to 80%. They additionally found that a volume of residual tumor remaining of less than 10 mL was predictive of longer OS. Therefore, when one counsels patients with diffuse and deep-seated tumors, an extent of resection threshold of 80% and volume of residual less than 10 mL are commonly thought to represent the mark needed to be of therapeutic benefit to individual patients. Although similar other retrospective studies have yielded comparable results, greater insight is needed in light of the WHO 2016 subclassification of WHO 2 gliomas (see later discussion).

WHO 2 gliomas may be difficult to visualize intraoperatively, and surgical adjuvants (see Todd Hollon and colleagues' article, "Surgical Adjuncts to Increase Extent of Resection: Intraoperative MRI, Fluorescence, and Raman Histology," in this issue), such as fluorescence-guided surgery, stimulated Raman histology, and intraoperative MRI, are not readily available across all centers treating patients. Therefore, it is important to understand the literature with respect to reoperation for residual or recurrent WHO 2 gliomas. Martino and colleagues[38] illustrated safety of reoperation for low-grade gliomas. In this study, the median time between operations was 4.1 years, and all patients remained alive over the median follow-up period of 6.6 years. The majority (58%) of patients had progressed to high-grade histology; one of the strongest predictors of OS was maximal GTR.

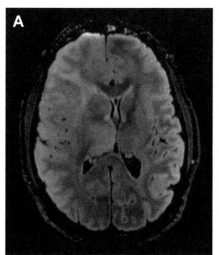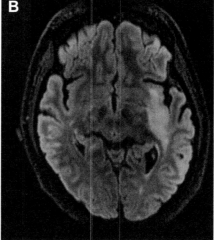

Fig. 1. Focal versus diffuse low-grade gliomas. WHO 2 gliomas may present either as diffuse tumors (*A*) similar to this illustrative case in which FLAIR signal encompasses the right frontal lobe, thalamus, and cingulate gyrus or focal tumors (*B*) as illustrated by FLAIR signal confined to the posterior left insula.

CONSIDERING THE EVIDENCE IN SUPPORT OF EXTENT OF RESECTION IN LIGHT OF MOLECULARLY SUBCLASSIFIED LOW GRADE GLIOMAS

Recently, the WHO classification of gliomas was updated based on molecular markers, which offers more precise prognostication and prediction of treatment response.[39] Gliomas are therefore classified using a layered diagnosis according to histologic as well as molecular criteria into astrocytomas and oligodendrogliomas. Molecular and genetic data supplements rather than displaces histologic classification. Layer 1 represents the final integrated diagnosis; layer 2 is the histologic classification; layer 3 designates WHO grade; and layer 4 allows for integration of molecular information. Integration of all 4 layers results in a single diagnostic entity describing the tumor with sufficient clarity to permit prognostication. We are only now beginning to understand how extent of tumor burden following surgery plays into this classification scheme. The definition of WHO 2 astrocytoma and oligodendroglioma is influenced heavily by the presence of IDH 1 and 2 mutations and balanced translocation of the p arm of chromosome 1 with the q arm of chromosome 19 (1p/19q codeletion). Oligodendrogliomas carry both IDH mutation and 1p19q codeletions.

Conversely, astrocytomas never contain 1p19q codeletions and are subdivided based on the presence or absence of IDH 1 or 2 mutations (Fig. 2). The previously popular oligoastrocytoma is now discouraged, used only used when IDH mutation and 1p/19q codeletion testing has either failed or is not possible. The distinction between astrocytomas and oligodendrogliomas (which harbor IDH 1 or 2 mutations and 1p19q codeletion) is clinically important, particularly because WHO 2 and 3 oligodendrogliomas treated with radiation therapy followed by procarbazine, lomustine, and vincristine have significantly lengthier survival compared with astrocytomas.[40]

It is important to appreciate that a molecular subclassification of gliomas can only be made following surgical resection. Even so, as advanced molecular imaging technologies improve, prospective understanding of glioma subtype may become available. Questions remain regarding the role of maximal extent of resection when considering molecularly favorable oligodendrogliomas in comparison to less favorable infiltrative astrocytomas, with and without IDH mutations (see Victoria E. Clark and Daniel P. Cahill's article, "EOR Versus Molecular Classification: What Matters When?," in this issue). There are some data available to date. Kawaguchi and

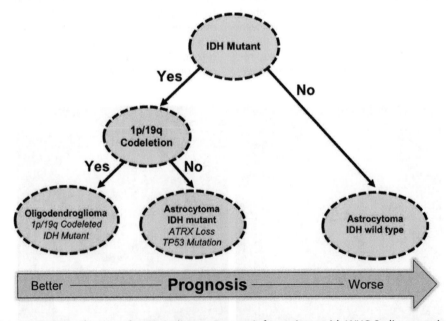

Fig. 2. Molecular subclassification of WHO 2 gliomas. Prognosis for patients with WHO 2 gliomas varies based on IDH mutation and 1p19q codeletion. Oligodendrogliomas are defined molecularly by the presence of 1p/19q codeletion with IDH 1 or 2 mutations. Astrocytomas are defined molecularly by IDH 1 or 2 mutations without 1p/19q codeletion and often have ATRX loss and TP53 mutation. IDH mutant astrocytomas have a more favorable prognosis. Astrocytomas without IDH mutations (IDH wild type) have the least favorable prognosis often comparable with glioblastoma.

colleagues[41] examined the impact of GTR versus non-gross total resection (non-GTR) on clinical outcomes within 3 molecular subtypes of WHO grade 3 gliomas: IDH 1/2 mutation with 1p/19q codeletion, IDH 1/2 mutation without 1p/19q codeletion, and IDH 1/2 wild-type. Although GTR led to a longer median OS and PFS than non-GTR, GTR only had a significant impact on OS in patients with IDH1/2 mutations without 1p/19q codeletion (astrocytomas IDH-mut). No significant differences in survival were observed between GTR and non-GTR in patients with molecularly unfavorable IDH 1/2 wild-type astrocytomas or IDH 1/2 mutation with 1p/19q codeletion oligodendrogliomas.[30] Focusing on extent of resection across molecular subtypes, univariate analysis suggested that smaller postoperative volume of residual disease was associated with greater OS in astrocytoma IDH mutant patients but only demonstrated a trend toward significance within oligodendroglioma patients. In patients with IDH-mutant astrocytomas, a postoperative tumor volume of less than 25 cm^3 was associated with longer overall compared with residual volumes greater than 25 cm^3.[30]

Cahill and colleagues[42] similarly found that the prognostic significance of extent of resection differed in WHO 3 anaplastic astrocytomas based on their IDH1 status. After examining EOR in 157 patients with anaplastic astrocytomas and 250 patients with GBM, the investigators reported that volume of residual enhancing tissue was associated with shorter OS in IDH1 wild-type tumors. Patel and colleagues[29] conducted a retrospective analysis of 74 patients with WHO 2 gliomas and known IDH mutational status. The effect of predictor variables on MPFS and OS was analyzed. Although the sample size was limited, this study yielded interesting results. Increasing EOR offered a survival benefit when considering the entire study population; however, stratifying by IDH status demonstrated that greater EOR independently extended MPFS and OS for IDH wild-type patients but not for patients identified as IDH mutant. It should be noted that the median follow-up period for this study was 3.7 years, and therefore, patients with molecularly favorable IDH mutant gliomas might experience the survival benefit of maximal resection in later years.[29] All published studies to date are limited by small sample sizes and relatively short follow-up periods, leaving much to be answered about this important topic. Taken together, the published literature highlights the idea that differences in clinical outcomes across subgroups suggest independent associations between extent of glioma resection based on molecular subtype.

BALANCING EXTENT OF RESECTION WITH FUNCTIONAL OUTCOMES: EVALUATING EOR DATA IN LIGHT OF AN EVOLVING UNDERSTANDING OF CORTICAL PLASTICITY

The evidence in support of maximal resection must be balanced alongside functional outcomes, particularly with respect to mobility, language, and nonlanguage cognitive domains. Functional performance is the driving force behind maintaining a maximal health-related quality of life (HRQOL), and these measures go beyond Karnofsky Performance Status. Preservation of quality of life is critically important and is thought to have an impact on survival. Long-term language outcomes following direct cortical and subcortical stimulation mapping of dominant hemisphere gliomas has been evaluated by several large clinical series (WHO grades 2-4).[43–45] During the immediate postoperative period, language temporarily worsens in 14% to 50% of patients.[44–46] One month following surgery, 78% to 100% of patients will have return of language to baseline preoperative function.[44,45] However, after 3 to 6 months, only 0% to 2.4% of patients will have worsened language function, and by and large, many patients are satisfied with their functional outcomes.[44,45] Long-term motor outcomes have similarly been examined in a retrospective analysis of 294 patients with gliomas found within the perirolandic region following intraoperative motor mapping.[47] Twenty percent of patients experienced a new postoperative motor deficit immediately following surgery; however, 58% recovered to their preoperative baseline within 1 month. Persistent motor deficits after 3 months were noted in 4.8% of patients, and this occurrence was highest when the corticospinal tract was identified during the resection.[47]

Working memory, attention, and executive functions significantly impact quality of life and are impacted by 3 evolving factors: (1) tumor location and infiltration patterns, (2) cytoreduction surgery, and (3) chemoradiation timing, dose, and frequency. An estimated 92% of glioma patients report impairments of cognition or mood at presentation.[48] Following surgery, 55% of patients had at least transient cognitive impairments primarily involving executive function, memory, and selective attention.[48–51] The extent to which functional impairments influence survival has been understudied in WHO 2 glioma patients. However, there are some data available to influence clinical decision making. McGirt and colleagues[52] retrospectively reviewed 1215 patients who underwent surgery for WHO 3 and 4 gliomas. Both preoperative motor and language dysfunction were assessed, although these assessments were not outlined in detailed. The presence of preoperative motor and language deficits both correlated with shorter OS following primary resection for both WHO 3 and 4 gliomas.[52]

Frequent or intractable seizures can be a major concern for glioma patients and negatively influences HRQOL. The ability to achieve seizure control is one of the most important factors in maintaining optimal quality of life.[53] A recent analysis of seizure control was conducted in 1181 epilepsy patients after subtotal or gross total lesionectomy. In addition, anatomically tailored resection of mesial and neocortical temporal structures combined with glioma resection was compared with glioma resection alone.[54] In that study, an estimated 43% of patients were seizure free after subtotal glioma resection, 79% were seizure free after gross total tumor resection, and 87% were seizure free after glioma resection with hippocampectomy and/or temporal neocortical resection.[54] It is therefore routinely accepted that greater extent of resection offers not only a survival benefit but also better seizure control in patients with low- or high-grade glioma.[54] There had been concern that cortical trauma caused by surgical resection of incidentally found low-grade glioma might increase the risk of developing epilepsy. However, it has been shown that the rate of perioperative seizures after glioma surgery is 0% to 3%, with 9.5% of patients developing seizures 3.2 to 6.5 years after surgery due to tumor progression.[55]

Cortical plasticity is the ability of the brain to change in response to experience, learning, or disease. It is an inherent feature of the brain that allows for the development and maintenance of nervous system function.[56] Cortical plasticity manifests itself through several physiologic mechanisms at the microscopic and macroscopic level. These processes include complex interactions, such as neurotransmitter receptor modulation and gliogenesis.[57,58] It is critical as glioma surgeons to balance maximal safe resection and functional postoperative outcomes following cytoreduction surgery, with the perspective of a "hodotopical" connectomal framework, not a localizationist view. A greater knowledge of how the adult brain changes in the setting of acute and chronic disease is fundamental to understanding the clinical course of neurologic conditions, including glioma. Several studies have studied cortical plasticity and clinical recovery in the setting of gliomas using noninvasive strategies.[43,59–64]

The recurrent nature of glioma has provided an opportunity to longitudinally study cortical and subcortical motor and cognitive functions using direct stimulation mapping. Intraoperative direct cortical mapping therefore offers an opportunity to study patients who sometimes undergo a second surgery in which direct electrical stimulation mapping is performed in the same brain region. In these instances, repeat direct electrical stimulation mapping provides a unique opportunity to directly and longitudinally examine whether cortical function reorganizes in the setting of disease. Southwell and colleagues[58] recently published data illustrating that changes in direct cortical mapping of language and motor sites were identified in 33.3% of subjects, and of 117 cortical sites tested, 1.1% experienced a gain of function and 40.9% experienced a loss of function between mapping intervals. The ability to predict and even encourage cortical plasticity would be clinically advantageous. A more complete understanding of cortical plasticity currently influences clinical decision making, because low-grade gliomas that infiltrate areas of functional significance may intentionally receive a subtotal resection with preservation of functional sites.[65] At recurrence, patients undergo repeat language and motor mapping, which often permits a more complete resection due to reorganization of functional areas.[58,65] The evidence in support of this staged approach to maximal resection is in the early stages. Much of these data has been derived from noninvasive and indirect measurements of brain function, such as functional MRI, PET, and transcranial magnetic stimulation. These data must now be reinterpreted in light of glioma molecular subclassification.

SUMMARY

Low-grade gliomas are a major cause of morbidity and mortality in the United States. Low-grade gliomas have a 10-year survival of 91% when extent of resection is greater than 90%. The impact of surgery based on molecular subclassification is currently under investigation. Functional language, motor, and cognitive status may be influenced by cortical plasticity. Therefore, the evidence in support of extent of resection must be balanced against a growing understanding of how gliomas influence connectomal networks.

REFERENCES

1. Barnholtz-Sloan JS, Sloan AE, Schwartz AG. Chapter 25: cancer of the brain and other central nervous system. In: Ries L, Young J, Keel G, et al, editors. SEER survival monograph: cancer survival among adults: U.S. SEER program, 1988-2001, patient and tumor characteristics. Bethesda (MD): National Cancer Institute; 2007. p. 203–14.

2. Lacroix M, Abi-Said D, Fourney DR, et al. A multivariate analysis of 416 patients with glioblastoma multiforme: prognosis, extent of resection, and survival. J Neurosurg 2001;95(2):190–8.

3. Lote K, Egeland T, Hager B, et al. Survival, prognostic factors, and therapeutic efficacy in low-grade glioma: a retrospective study in 379 patients. J Clin Oncol 1997;15(9):3129–40.

4. Nakamura M, Konishi N, Tsunoda S, et al. Analysis of prognostic and survival factors related to treatment of low-grade astrocytomas in adults. Oncology 2000;58(2):108–16.

5. Nicolato A, Gerosa MA, Fina P, et al. Prognostic factors in low-grade supratentorial astrocytomas: a uni-multivariate statistical analysis in 76 surgically treated adult patients. Surg Neurol 1995;44(3): 208–21 [discussion: 221–3].

6. Scerrati M, Roselli R, Iacoangeli M, et al. Prognostic factors in low grade (WHO grade II) gliomas of the cerebral hemispheres: the role of surgery. J Neurol Neurosurg Psychiatry 1996;61(3):291–6.

7. Yan H, Parsons DW, Jin G, et al. IDH1 and IDH2 mutations in gliomas. N Engl J Med 2009;360(8): 765–73.

8. Yordanova YN, Duffau H. Supratotal resection of diffuse gliomas - an overview of its multifaceted implications. Neurochirurgie 2017;63(3):243–9.

9. Bauman G, Pahapill P, Macdonald D, et al. Low grade glioma: a measuring radiographic response to radiotherapy. Can J Neurol Sci 1999;26(1):18–22.

10. Claus EB, Horlacher A, Hsu L, et al. Survival rates in patients with low-grade glioma after intraoperative magnetic resonance image guidance. Cancer 2005;103(6):1227–33.

11. Hollon T, Nguyen V, Smith BW, et al. Supratentorial hemispheric ependymomas: an analysis of 109 adults for survival and prognostic factors. J Neurosurg 2016;8:1–9.

12. Incekara F, Olubiyi O, Ozdemir A, et al. The value of pre- and intraoperative adjuncts on the extent of resection of hemispheric low-grade gliomas: a retrospective analysis. J Neurol Surg A Cent Eur Neurosurg 2016;77(2):79–87.

13. Ito S, Chandler KL, Prados MD, et al. Proliferative potential and prognostic evaluation of low-grade astrocytomas. J Neurooncol 1994;19(1):1–9.

14. Johannesen TB, Langmark F, Lote K. Progress in long-term survival in adult patients with supratentorial low-grade gliomas: a population-based study of 993 patients in whom tumors were diagnosed between 1970 and 1993. J Neurosurg 2003;99(5): 854–62.

15. Karim AB, Maat B, Hatlevoll R, et al. A randomized trial on dose-response in radiation therapy of low-grade cerebral glioma: European Organization for Research and Treatment of Cancer (EORTC) Study 22844. Int J Radiat Oncol Biol Phys 1996;36(3):549–56.

16. Leighton C, Fisher B, Bauman G, et al. Supratentorial low-grade glioma in adults: an analysis of prognostic factors and timing of radiation. J Clin Oncol 1997;15(4):1294–301.

17. North CA, North RB, Epstein JA, et al. Low-grade cerebral astrocytomas. Survival and quality of life after radiation therapy. Cancer 1990;66(1):6–14.

18. Peraud A, Ansari H, Bise K, et al. Clinical outcome of supratentorial astrocytoma WHO grade II. Acta Neurochir 1998;140(12):1213–22.

19. Philippon JH, Clemenceau SH, Fauchon FH, et al. Supratentorial low-grade astrocytomas in adults. Neurosurgery 1993;32(4):554–9.

20. Rajan B, Pickuth D, Ashley S, et al. The management of histologically unverified presumed cerebral gliomas with radiotherapy. Int J Radiat Oncol Biol Phys 1994;28(2):405–13.

21. Sanai N, Berger MS. Glioma extent of resection and its impact on patient outcome. Neurosurgery 2008; 62(4):753–64 [discussion: 264–6].

22. Shaw E, Arusell R, Scheithauer B, et al. Prospective randomized trial of low- versus high-dose radiation therapy in adults with supratentorial low-grade glioma: initial report of a North Central Cancer Treatment Group/Radiation Therapy Oncology Group/Eastern Cooperative Oncology Group study. J Clin Oncol 2002;20(9):2267–76.

23. Shibamoto Y, Kitakabu Y, Takahashi M, et al. Supratentorial low-grade astrocytoma. Correlation of computed tomography findings with effect of radiation therapy and prognostic variables. Cancer 1993; 72(1):190–5.

24. Smith JS, Chang EF, Lamborn KR, et al. Role of extent of resection in the long-term outcome of low-grade hemispheric gliomas. J Clin Oncol 2008; 26(8):1338–45.

25. Snyder LA, Wolf AB, Oppenlander ME, et al. The impact of extent of resection on malignant transformation of pure oligodendrogliomas. J Neurosurg 2014;120(2):309–14.

26. van Veelen ML, Avezaat CJ, Kros JM, et al. Supratentorial low grade astrocytoma: prognostic factors, dedifferentiation, and the issue of early versus late surgery. J Neurol Neurosurg Psychiatry 1998;64(5): 581–7.

27. Whitton AC, Bloom HJ. Low grade glioma of the cerebral hemispheres in adults: a retrospective analysis of 88 cases. Int J Radiat Oncol Biol Phys 1990;18(4):783–6.

28. Yeh SA, Ho JT, Lui CC, et al. Treatment outcomes and prognostic factors in patients with supratentorial low-grade gliomas. Br J Radiol 2005;78(927):230–5.

29. Patel T, Bander ED, Venn RA, et al. The role of extent of resection in IDH1 wild-type or mutant low-grade gliomas. Neurosurgery 2018;82(6):808–14.

30. Wijnenga MMJ, French PJ, Dubbink HJ, et al. The impact of surgery in molecularly defined low-grade

glioma: an integrated clinical, radiological, and molecular analysis. Neuro Oncol 2018;20(1):103–12.

31. Pekmezci M, Rice T, Molinaro AM, et al. Adult infiltrating gliomas with WHO 2016 integrated diagnosis: additional prognostic roles of ATRX and TERT. Acta Neuropathol 2017;133(6):1001–16.

32. Jakola AS, Myrmel KS, Kloster R, et al. Comparison of a strategy favoring early surgical resection vs a strategy favoring watchful waiting in low-grade gliomas. JAMA 2012;308(18):1881–8.

33. Pallud J, Fontaine D, Duffau H, et al. Natural history of incidental World Health Organization grade II gliomas. Ann Neurol 2010;68(5):727–33.

34. Potts MB, Smith JS, Molinaro AM, et al. Natural history and surgical management of incidentally discovered low-grade gliomas. J Neurosurg 2012; 116(2):365–72.

35. Frazier JL, Johnson MW, Burger PC, et al. Rapid malignant transformation of low-grade astrocytomas: report of 2 cases and review of the literature. World Neurosurg 2010;73(1):53–62 [discussion: e5].

36. Piepmeier J, Christopher S, Spencer D, et al. Variations in the natural history and survival of patients with supratentorial low-grade astrocytomas. Neurosurgery 1996;38(5):872–8.

37. Recht LD, Lew R, Smith TW. Suspected low-grade glioma: is deferring treatment safe? Ann Neurol 1992;31(4):431–6.

38. Martino J, Taillandier L, Moritz-Gasser S, et al. Reoperation is a safe and effective therapeutic strategy in recurrent WHO grade II gliomas within eloquent areas. Acta Neurochir (Wien) 2009;151(5):427–36 [discussion: 436].

39. Louis DN, Perry A, Reifenberger G, et al. The 2016 World Health Organization classification of tumors of the central nervous system: a summary. Acta Neuropathol 2016;131(6):803–20.

40. Buckner JC, Shaw EG, Pugh SL, et al. Radiation plus Procarbazine, CCNU, and Vincristine in Low-Grade Glioma. N Engl J Med 2016;374(14): 1344–55.

41. Kawaguchi T, Sonoda Y, Shibahara I, et al. Impact of gross total resection in patients with WHO grade III glioma harboring the IDH 1/2 mutation without the 1p/19q co-deletion. J Neurooncol 2016;129(3): 505–14.

42. Cahill DP, Beiko J, Suki D, et al. IDH1 status and survival benefit from surgical resection of enhancing and nonenhancing tumor in malignant astrocytomas. J Clin Oncol 2012;30(15_suppl):2019.

43. Duffau H, Capelle L, Denvil D, et al. Functional recovery after surgical resection of low grade gliomas in eloquent brain: hypothesis of brain compensation. J Neurol Neurosurg Psychiatry 2003;74(7):901–7.

44. Duffau H, Moritz-Gasser S, Gatignol P. Functional outcome after language mapping for insular World Health Organization Grade II gliomas in the dominant hemisphere: experience with 24 patients. Neurosurg Focus 2009;27(2):E7.

45. Sanai N, Mirzadeh Z, Berger MS. Functional outcome after language mapping for glioma resection. N Engl J Med 2008;358(1):18–27.

46. Wilson SM, Lam D, Babiak MC, et al. Transient aphasias after left hemisphere resective surgery. J Neurosurg 2015;123(3):581–93.

47. Keles GE, Lundin DA, Lamborn KR, et al. Intraoperative subcortical stimulation mapping for hemispherical perirolandic gliomas located within or adjacent to the descending motor pathways: evaluation of morbidity and assessment of functional outcome in 294 patients. J Neurosurg 2004;100(3):369–75.

48. Racine CA, Li J, Molinaro AM, et al. Neurocognitive function in newly diagnosed low-grade glioma patients undergoing surgical resection with awake mapping techniques. Neurosurgery 2015;77(3):371–9.

49. Douw L, Klein M, Fagel SS, et al. Cognitive and radiological effects of radiotherapy in patients with low-grade glioma: long-term follow-up. Lancet Neurol 2009;8(9):810–8.

50. Taphoorn MJ, Klein M. Cognitive deficits in adult patients with brain tumours. Lancet Neurol 2004;3(3): 159–68.

51. Ahmadi R, Dictus C, Hartmann C, et al. Long-term outcome and survival of surgically treated supratentorial low-grade glioma in adult patients. Acta Neurochir (Wien) 2009;151(11):1359–65.

52. McGirt MJ, Chaichana KL, Gathinji M, et al. Independent association of extent of resection with survival in patients with malignant brain astrocytoma. J Neurosurg 2009;110(1):156–62.

53. Ruda R, Bello L, Duffau H, et al. Seizures in low-grade gliomas: natural history, pathogenesis, and outcome after treatments. Neuro Oncol 2012; 14(Suppl 4):iv55–64.

54. Englot DJ, Han SJ, Berger MS, et al. Extent of surgical resection predicts seizure freedom in low-grade temporal lobe brain tumors. Neurosurgery 2012; 70(4):921–8.

55. de Oliveira Lima GL, Duffau H. Is there a risk of seizures in "preventive" awake surgery for incidental diffuse low-grade gliomas? J Neurosurg 2015; 122(6):1397–405.

56. Pascual-Leone A, Amedi A, Fregni F, et al. The plastic human brain cortex. Annu Rev Neurosci 2005;28: 377–401.

57. Duffau H. Brain plasticity: from pathophysiological mechanisms to therapeutic applications. J Clin Neurosci 2006;13(9):885–97.

58. Southwell DG, Hervey-Jumper SL, Perry DW, et al. Intraoperative mapping during repeat awake craniotomy reveals the functional plasticity of adult cortex. J Neurosurg 2015;6:1–10.

59. Duffau H, Denvil D, Capelle L. Long term reshaping of language, sensory, and motor maps after glioma

resection: a new parameter to integrate in the surgical strategy. J Neurol Neurosurg Psychiatry 2002; 72(4):511–6.

60. Fandino J, Kollias SS, Wieser HG, et al. Intraoperative validation of functional magnetic resonance imaging and cortical reorganization patterns in patients with brain tumors involving the primary motor cortex. J Neurosurg 1999;91(2):238–50.

61. Krieg SM, Sollmann N, Hauck T, et al. Repeated mapping of cortical language sites by preoperative navigated transcranial magnetic stimulation compared to repeated intraoperative DCS mapping in awake craniotomy. BMC Neurosci 2014;15:20.

62. Robles SG, Gatignol P, Lehericy S, et al. Long-term brain plasticity allowing a multistage surgical approach to World Health Organization Grade II

gliomas in eloquent areas. J Neurosurg 2008; 109(4):615–24.

63. Seitz RJ, Huang Y, Knorr U, et al. Large-scale plasticity of the human motor cortex. Neuroreport 1995; 6(5):742–4.

64. Wunderlich G, Knorr U, Herzog H, et al. Precentral glioma location determines the displacement of cortical hand representation. Neurosurgery 1998; 42(1):18–26.

65. Hervey-Jumper SL, Li J, Lau D, et al. Awake craniotomy to maximize glioma resection: methods and technical nuances over a 27-year period. J Neurosurg 2015;123(2):325–39.

66. Chaichana KL, Zadnik P, Weingart JD, et al. Multiple resections for patients with glioblastoma: prolonging survival. J Neurosurg 2013;118(4):812–20.

Extent of Resection Versus Molecular Classification
What Matters When?

Victoria E. Clark, MD, PhD, Daniel P. Cahill, MD, PhD*

KEYWORDS

- Low-grade gliomas • Extent of resection • Molecular classification • *IDH1* mutant
- Survival analysis

KEY POINTS

- Although the pathways underlying grade II diffuse gliomas are increasingly elucidated, there are no available targeted therapies leveraging this molecular knowledge available for clinical practice.
- In the interim, the available literature supports the application of adjunctive therapies (specifically, the combination of radiation therapy + PCV) after maximal safe resection to improve the overall survival of low-grade gliomas.
- The benefit of maximal safe resection is more pronounced in astrocytomas compared with oligodendrogliomas, which may be a reflection of their intrinsically more aggressive clinical course compared with oligodendrogliomas.

LOW-GRADE GLIOMAS: A DEFINITION IN TRANSITION
IDH1 Mutant Low-Grade Gliomas

For the purpose of this article, low-grade gliomas refers exclusively to World Health Organization (WHO) grade II diffuse astrocytic and oligodendroglial tumors (**Table 1**). These tumors are homogenous in terms of bearing the hallmark *IDH1/2* mutations and yet have striking variation in the propensity for malignant transformation. As summarized in detail elsewhere in this issue, WHO grade II astrocytomas are characterized by *IDH* gain-of-function mutations and loss of *TP53* and *ATRX*. The median age of diagnosis is 36 years old, with a median survival of 10.9 years.[1] WHO grade II oligodendrogliomas are genetically defined by *IDH* mutations, 1p/19q codeletions (frequently with *FUBP1* or *CIC* mutations), and activating *TERT* promoter mutations. The median age of diagnosis for this tumor is older (age 43 years)[2] with a median survival of 17.1 years.[3] Grade II oligoastrocytomas, a categorization treated by the WHO 2016 as more reflective of inadequate molecular testing, traditionally have been thought to have a survival intermediate between astrocytomas and oligodendrogliomas.

For both low-grade glioma lineages, the diagnostic *IDH1* neomorphic mutation generates the oncometabolite 2-HG, leading to dysregulation of histone lysine demethylase and ultimately global hypermethylation of CpG islands (G-CIMP).[4,5] The mechanism of malignant progression in *IDH1* mutant low-grade gliomas is an area of intensive study. An integrated genomic approach, including sequencing, copy number, expression, and DNA methylation data from patient-matched low-grade and progressed *IDH1* mutant gliomas, revealed

Disclosure Statement: Dr. Cahill received fund from Burroughs-Wellcome Fund # 1007616.02 NIH (CA P50 CA165962).
Department of Neurosurgery, Massachusetts General Hospital, 55 Fruit Street, Boston, MA 02114, USA
* Corresponding author.
E-mail address: cahill@mgh.harvard.edu

Table 1
Clinical and genetic characteristics of WHO grade II low-grade gliomas

	IDH Mutant		IDH Wild Type Can Generally Be Recategorized into Another WHO Tumor Type with Additional Molecular Testing
	Astrocytoma	Oligodendroglioma	
Age at diagnosis	Younger (median, age 36)	Older (median, age 44)	Intermediate (median, age 39.6)
Genetics	• TP53 mutations • ATRX mutations	• 1p/19q loss • FUBP1 mutations • CIC mutations • TERT promoter mutations	• Genetically heterogeneous • Subgroup matching IDH wt glioblastoma multiforme (EGFR amp, TERT promoter mutation); poor prognosis • Subgroup matching pediatric astrocytomas (BRAF V600E, MYB amplification); better prognosis
Median survival	10.9 y	17.1 y	Heterogeneous, per mutation (eg, TERT mutant- 1.76 y vs TERT wt- 10.65 y)
Impact of surgical resection on survival	Small degree of residual tumor negatively impacts survival	Small degree of residual tumor may not impact survival	Varies based on driver mutation

activation of Myc signaling, RTK-RAS-PI3K signaling, alterations in CDKN2A-CDKN2B, and increased methylation in embryonic targets of Polycomb repressive complex 2 (PRC2).[6]

IDH1 Wild-Type Low-Grade Gliomas

The subgroup of IDH1 wild-type diffuse glioma is treated as transitional by the WHO 2016 and recent studies reveal heterogeneity in the survival of patients with histologically low-grade diffuse astrocytomas but no detectable IDH1/2 mutations.[7–9] Molecularly, the majority of tumors in this group resemble glioblastoma despite a low-grade histologic appearance, although a smaller subset bear a genomic profile aligned with grade I astrocytomas (eg, pilocytic). In a study of 212 WHO grade II diffuse astrocytomas defined histologically, all 25 of the noncontrast enhancing, truly IDH1/2 wild-type (by sequencing) tumors could be reclassified using a combination of sequencing, methylation profiling, and copy number profiling into glioblastoma multiforme, diffuse midline glioma with H3K27M mutation, pilocytic astrocytoma, or normal brain tissue.[7] In this study, 0 of 25 IDH1 wild-type, with a histologic appearance consistent with diffuse low-grade gliomas could not be reclassified into another tumor type. This finding is consistent with the findings of Poulen and colleagues,[8] where a subset of the 31 "IDH1

wt" grade II astrocytomas had a median survival of 3.5 years, whereas others had a 5-year survival of 77%. Additional work by Aibaidula and colleagues[9] of 168 IDH1 wt grade II and III gliomas demonstrated that these tumors could be grouped into molecularly high grade and molecularly low grade, irrespective of histologic grade, which bore molecular hallmarks characteristic of primary glioblastoma multiforme (molecularly high grade) or characteristic of pediatric diffuse low-grade gliomas (molecularly low grade), which tended to occur in younger adults and may reflect the true extension of pediatric low-grade gliomas.

EXTENT OF RESECTION AND THE IMPACT ON SURVIVAL

Any discussion regarding the impact of the extent of resection (EOR) on improving survival, malignant progression, and/or quality of life in patients with low-grade gliomas must begin with the acknowledgment that there are no randomized, controlled trials evaluating these clinical questions.[10] Part of the challenge in combining studies from the available literature into metaanalyses includes variations in the precision of the classification and measurement of the degree of surgical resection. For example, the scale of resection is treated by some studies as binary (eg, resection vs biopsy), whereas other studies use sophisticated MRI volumetrics characteristics based on fluid-attenuated inversion recovery to quantify the EOR, creating difficulties in direct comparisons between studies. Complicating this also is timing of surgical resection—a short-term "watch and wait" strategy followed by complete resection may not negatively impact survival compared with upfront complete resection, but the time of observation may be affected by the baseline aggressiveness of the tumor (eg, more aggressive tumors progress earlier and are resected earlier). Additionally, available studies are not uniform in terms of postoperative management; for example, EOR studies are not controlled for adjuvant chemotherapy or radiation therapy, both of which may affect survival, progression, and cognition. Furthermore, the new WHO diagnostics reclassify the very definition of WHO grade II gliomas, with oligodendrogliomas as defined by *IDH1*/1p-19q codeletions having intrinsically better survival compared with astrocytomas as defined by *IDH1/ATRX/TP53* mutations (see **Table 1**). Previous studies lacking these molecular distinctions are fundamentally susceptible to sample bias, and there is no way to control and stratify for mutational underpinning in nonrandomized studies that have compared maximal EOR versus biopsy. Additionally, there is evidence that tumor size at the time of diagnosis portends a worse prognosis, regardless of the degree of resection achieved,[11] and these tumors are also less likely to undergo true gross total resection (GTR) as a technical limitation.

With these caveats, several lines of evidence support maximal safe resection over biopsy alone or waiting for radiographic progression. In a study by Jakola and colleagues,[12] the outcomes between 2 hospitals in Norway, one that tended to biopsy and then observe (71% of the time) and the other which tended to proceed with early resection (86% of the time), were compared. The hospital that tended to proceed with early resection had significantly better overall survival (OS) compared with the hospital that preferred biopsy and watchful waiting ($P = .01$), with expected 7-year survivals of 68% versus 44%, respectively. When considering tumors that underwent biopsy at the hospital where biopsy was preferred and compared with craniotomy at the hospital where craniotomy was preferred, the median survival was 5.8 years for the biopsy group, but the median survival was not reached at hospital B. This study was updated in 2017 to take into account the new WHO classification of low-grade glioma, at which point the median survival for the craniotomy group at hospital B was 14.4 years and the group treated at hospital B had

better survival regardless of mutational profile.[13] However, there are clear methodologic limitations to this study, including a lack of randomization and lack of data on the EOR, as well as a lack of data on postoperative treatment modalities (chemotherapy/radiation therapy).

In a study by Smith and colleagues,[11] a series of 216 adult low-grade gliomas resected from 1989 to 2005 revealed that, after adjusting for age, Karnofsky Performance Score (KPS), tumor histology, and tumor location, tumors with at least 90% EOR (as defined by volumetric analysis of reduction of fluid-attenuated inversion recovery on postoperative MRI) had 5- and 8-year OS rates of 97% and 91%, respectively. In contrast, patients with less than 90% EOR had 5- and 8-year OS rates of 76% and 60%, respectively. As a caveat, the tumors that had greater than 90% resection tended to have a smaller preoperative volume, which may reflect differences in the underlying biology. Related to this, regardless of the EOR, tumors with a greater preoperative volume had statistically worse OS (hazard ratio, 4.442; $P = .004$) as well as worse progression-free survival (hazard ratio, 2.711; $P<.001$). Additionally, the subset of patients who received radiation therapy and/or chemotherapy after surgical resection (true for a subset of subtotally resected tumors) were combined in the analysis with the patients who did not.

A recent metaanalysis argued for a gradient of improved 5- and 10-year survival rates, with patients undergoing GTR having an improved survival compared with patients who underwent subtotal resection (STR), and patients with STR having an improved survival over patients who underwent biopsy alone.[14] This analysis, which mainly combined retrospective studies published in 1990s, showed that the 5-year survival rate for patients with low-grade glioma was significantly higher in patients undergoing GTR compared with STR (odds ratio [OR], 3.90; 16 studies, 1328 cases) as well as to biopsy (OR, 5.43; 9 studies, 775 cases). A metaanalysis of 11 studies (1147 cases) showed that patients undergoing STR compared with biopsy had a significantly higher 5-year survival rates (OR, 1.75). This study also found that the 10-year survival rate for patients with low-grade glioma was higher in patients undergoing GTR compared with STR (OR, 7.91; 11 studies, 907 cases), GTR compared with biopsy (OR, 10.17; 5 studies, 186 cases), and STR compared with biopsy (OR, 2.21; 6 studies, 408 cases). Flaws associated with this analysis include the mix of adjuvant therapies that the patients underwent, as well as the nonstandardized definition of EOR between studies. For example, the majority of the included studies either did not specify how

EOR was determined or relied on the operative report or surgeon's description instead of objective postoperative imaging characteristics. Additionally, the preoperative volume of the tumors were not considered, so there is possible confounding between the preoperative size of the tumors and the extent that was able to be resected (eg, the largest tumors were unable to undergo GTR and also had worse outcomes).

SUPRATOTAL RESECTION

A biopsy study of 101 stereotactic biopsies (64 within regions of radiographic abnormalities, 37 from outside the regions of radiographic abnormalities) from 16 patients for diffuse low-grade oligodendrogliomas revealed isolated tumor cells up to 20 mm beyond radiographic evidence of tumor per MRI.[15] To test whether supratotal resection (removing the fluid-attenuated inversion recovery abnormality as well as an additional margin) of diffuse low-grade gliomas would provide superior outcomes, the rates of malignant transformation and recurrence were compared between patients undergoing supratotal resection versus GTR.[16] Using awake functional stimulation to define functional boundaries, supratotal resection was achieved in 15 patients with low-grade gliomas. For these patients, there were no instances of malignant transformation over an average of 35.7 months of postoperative follow-up and tumor recurrence was observed in 4 of 15 patients (average time to recurrence, 38 months). In contrast, a control group of 29 patients who underwent GTR had anaplastic transformation in 7 cases. In a study with more extensive follow-up (mean follow-up, 132 months), Duffau[17] studied the clinical outcomes of 16 patients who underwent awake surgery with intraoperative stimulation to define the functional boundaries of resection. None of the tumors underwent malignant transformation, none of the patients died during the time of follow-up, and only 8 of the tumors recurred (average, 70.3 months; see Hugues Duffau's article, "Higher Order Surgical Questions for Diffuse Low-Grade Gliomas: Supramaximal Resection, Neuroplasticity and Screening," in this issue). In combination, these studies suggest a rationale for and potential benefit to supratotal resection to delay malignant transformation of low-grade glioma; however, studies with larger sample sizes are needed.

EXTENT OF RESECTION AND MOLECULAR SUBTYPING

More recent EOR studies have used molecular definitions of grades II and III gliomas and have suggested differences in the impact of maximal resection in astrocytomas versus oligodendrogliomas (see **Table 1**). For grade III anaplastic astrocytomas (defined as *IDH* mutant, 1p/19q retained), patients who underwent GTR had statistically significant improved survival (*P* = .005).[18] However, for grade III anaplastic oligodendrogliomas (defined as *IDH* mutant, 1p/19q codeletion), there was no significant survival difference in patients who underwent GTR versus STR (*P* = .14). This pattern was also reflected in a later analysis comparing the survival benefit granted by the EOR in grade II astrocytomas (*IDH1* mutant, 1p/19q retained) versus grade II oligodendrogliomas (*IDH1* mutant, 1p/19q codeleted).[19] In this study, a residual volume of 0.1 to 5.0 cm^3 for grade II astrocytomas granted a significantly worse OS compared with GTR; however, even up to 25 cm^3 of residual tumor had a significantly better OS compared with greater than 25 cm^3. In contrast, there was no significant improvement in the survival of grade II oligodendrogliomas in patients with GTR versus small residual tumor (0.1–5.0 cm^3).

EXTENT OF RESECTION AND QUALITY OF LIFE

Regardless of the EOR, patients with low-grade gliomas survive on the scale of years; therefore, quality of life metrics are important endpoints for clinical consideration. In a retrospective study by Chang and colleagues,[20] 81% of patients (269/332) with low-grade gliomas presented with seizures, and 49% of these patients (132/269) had medication-refractory epilepsy. At both 6 and 12 months, 91% of patients who presented with seizures had at least meaningful improvement (Engel class I–III) in their seizure control postoperatively. Of patients who presented with seizures, 67% had no seizures at 6 and 12 months of follow-up after resection, including approximately 50% of patients who presented with medication-refractory epilepsy. GTR was significantly associated with freedom from seizures (OR, 16; *P* = .0064) and a preoperative seizure history of more than 1 year was associated with worse postoperative seizure control (OR, 0.285; *P* = .003). This finding argues for early and aggressive surgical intervention for patients with low-grade gliomas presenting with seizures.

Similarly, in a study of low-grade gliomas of the insula, all of the 52 patients analyzed presented with seizures.[21] An analysis of postoperative seizure control and the EOR by volumetric analysis using preoperative and postoperative MRI demonstrated that increased EOR was associated with increased rate of achieving Engel class I (seizure free). The rate of Engel class I in patients with more than 90% EOR was 85.71%; for patients with an EOR of 70% to 89%, the rate was 65.22% and it was 0% for patients with less than a 70% EOR. Ultimately, however, on multivariate analysis EOR was not associated with improved seizure control and the only factor significantly impacting postoperative seizure control was a quantification of how diffuse the tumor's growth pattern (as defined by preoperative increased delta VT2T1 value), which also had a negative association with EOR.

In addition to seizure control, whether surgery improves or harms cognitive function in patients with low-grade glioma is another important consideration. Barzilai and colleagues[22] performed a retrospective analysis of 49 patients with low-grade gliomas (including a subset of pilocytic astrocytomas and gangliogliomas) who underwent full neurocognitive testing before and after attempting maximal safe resection. At baseline, the 49 patients had normal intelligence and abstract thinking but showed significant impairment in memory ($z = -4.03$). For the 26 dominant-sided tumors (mean EOR of 76% by volumetrics), there was a significant improvement in memory and executive function. For the 23 nondominant sided tumors (mean EOR of 83%), there was a significant improvement in memory only after attempted maximal safe resection. The caveats to this study include a lack of comparison of cognitive improvement to patients undergoing biopsy alone, and the heterogeneity of tumors pooled together (eg, only 29 of the 48 patients included were mutated for *IDH1*).

MOLECULAR CLASSIFICATION AND NOVEL THERAPEUTICS

These studies suggest a benefit for maximal safe surgical resection of low-grade gliomas, an effect that seems to be more striking for grade II astrocytomas compared with grade II oligodendrogliomas.

For the tumors that cannot be safely resected or that recur despite radiographic GTR, the identification of the molecular mechanisms driving low-grade glioma formation as well as malignant progression have fueled a field of active translational study for targeted adjuncts to surgical resection (**Fig. 1**).

There is an ongoing clinical trial for the use of 2-HG suppressors AG-120 or AG-881 in recurrent grade II or III confirmed *IDH1* mutant gliomas (NCT03343197). However, Johannessen and colleagues[23] demonstrate that, in a transformed astrocyte culture model, mutant *IDH1* is important in the initiation but not the maintenance of gliomagenesis and therapeutic targeting of mutant *IDH1* loses effectiveness after 4 days in their model.

Another approach capitalizes on the finding that 2HG creates a defect in homologous recombination, rendering *IDH1* mutant cell lines susceptible to PARP (poly(adenosine 5′-diphosphate–ribose) polymerase) inhibition.[24] There is currently a phase II clinical trial (NCT03212274) studying the PARP inhibitor olaparib in recurrent or progressive *IDH1/2* mutant gliomas as well as other *IDH1* mutant solid tumor types.

Another strategy focuses on reversing the G-CIMP hypermethylation phenotype associated with *IDH* mutations. Decitabine, a DNA methyltransferase inhibitor, was demonstrated to reverse the G-CIMP phenotype in vitro, resulting in the upregulation of glial differentiation genes and reduced cell growth in patient-derived *IDH1* mutant glioma cell lines.[25]

In addition to direct pharmacologic inhibition of *IDH1* or the perceived downstream effects (HR defects, G-CIMP), multiple clinical trials of immunotherapy with vaccines raised against the mutant epitope are currently recruiting. Schumacher and colleagues[26] demonstrated that an IDH1 R132H vaccine induced a Th-mediated immune response and reduced tumor growth in a humanized mouse model. Currently, there are 3

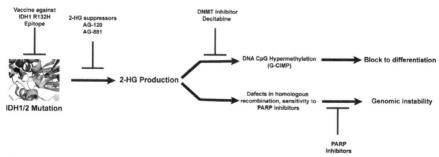

Fig. 1. Novel therapeutics target multiple steps in IDH-driven low-grade gliomagenesis. 2-HG, 2-hydroxyglutarate; CpG, 5′-cytosine-phosphate-guanine-3′; G-CIMP, glioma-CpG island methylator phenotype; PARP, poly ADP (adenosine diphosphate)-ribose polymerase.

phase I IDH1-specific immunotherapy trials underway, including the PEPIDH1M vaccine for grade II IDH1 mutant gliomas (recurrent or progressive, NCT02193347).

Because *IDH1* targeted therapy has not yet come to clinical fruition, the application of adjuvant radiation therapy and/or chemotherapy after surgery has been studied relative to the subgroups of low-grade gliomas, as defined by the 2016 WHO classification. A study by Buckner and colleagues[27] on patients with grade II gliomas (defined histologically, not by WHO 2016 mutational criteria) who had undergone STR or biopsy and were randomized to either radiation therapy alone or radiation therapy + PCV showed a survival benefit to all groups of grade II gliomas (oligodendrogliomas, astrocytomas, and oligoastrocytomas) that received both radiation therapy + PCV. A subgroup analysis of *IDH1* mutated tumors also demonstrated improved survival to the patients who underwent radiation therapy + PCV versus radiation therapy alone ($P = .02$). The median OS was 13.3 years for the combined group of low-grade gliomas who received radiation therapy + PCV compared with 7.8 years with radiation therapy alone ($P = .003$).

SUMMARY

Although the pathways underlying grade II diffuse gliomas are increasingly elucidated, there are unfortunately no available targeted therapies leveraging this molecular knowledge available for clinical practice. There are, however, multiple clinical trials underway that aim to exploit the class-defining neomorphic *IDH1* mutation to halt tumor progression. In the interim, the available literature supports the application of adjunctive therapies (specifically, the combination of radiation therapy + PCV) after maximal safe resection to improve the OS of low-grade gliomas. The benefit of maximal safe resection is more pronounced in astrocytomas, which may be a reflection of their intrinsically more aggressive clinical course compared with oligodendrogliomas.

REFERENCES

1. Reuss DE, Mamatjan Y, Schrimpf D, et al. IDH mutant diffuse and anaplastic astrocytomas have similar age at presentation and little difference in survival: a grading problem for WHO. Acta Neuropathol 2015;129(6):867–73.
2. Ostrom QT, Gittleman H, Liao P, et al. CBTRUS statistical report: primary brain and other central nervous system tumors diagnosed in the United States in 2010-2014. Neuro Oncol 2017;19(suppl_5):v1–88.
3. Killela PJ, Pirozzi CJ, Healy P, et al. Mutations in IDH1, IDH2, and in the TERT promoter define clinically distinct subgroups of adult malignant gliomas. Oncotarget 2014;5(6):1515–25.
4. Miller JJ, Shih HA, Andronesi OC, et al. Isocitrate dehydrogenase-mutant glioma: evolving clinical and therapeutic implications. Cancer 2017;123(23):4535–46.
5. Han CH, Batchelor TT. Isocitrate dehydrogenase mutation as a therapeutic target in gliomas. Chin Clin Oncol 2017;6(3):33.
6. Bai H, Harmanci AS, Erson-Omay EZ, et al. Integrated genomic characterization of IDH1-mutant glioma malignant progression. Nat Genet 2016;48(1):59–66.
7. Hasselblatt M, Jaber M, Reuss D, et al. Diffuse astrocytoma, IDH-wildtype: a dissolving diagnosis. J Neuropathol Exp Neurol 2018;77(6):422–5.
8. Poulen G, Goze C, Rigau V, et al. Huge heterogeneity in survival in a subset of adult patients with resected, wild-type isocitrate dehydrogenase status, WHO grade II astrocytomas. J Neurosurg 2018;1–10. [Epub ahead of print].
9. Aibaidula A, Chan AK, Shi Z, et al. Adult IDH wild-type lower-grade gliomas should be further stratified. Neuro Oncol 2017;19(10):1327–37.
10. Jiang B, Chaichana K, Veeravagu A, et al. Biopsy versus resection for the management of low-grade gliomas. Cochrane Database Syst Rev 2017;(4):CD009319.
11. Smith JS, Chang EF, Lamborn KR, et al. Role of extent of resection in the long-term outcome of low-grade hemispheric gliomas. J Clin Oncol 2008;26(8):1338–45.
12. Jakola AS, Myrmel KS, Kloster R, et al. Comparison of a strategy favoring early surgical resection vs a strategy favoring watchful waiting in low-grade gliomas. JAMA 2012;308(18):1881–8.
13. Jakola AS, Skjulsvik AJ, Myrmel KS, et al. Surgical resection versus watchful waiting in low-grade gliomas. Ann Oncol 2017;28(8):1942–8.
14. Xia L, Fang C, Chen G, et al. Relationship between the extent of resection and the survival of patients with low-grade gliomas: a systematic review and meta-analysis. BMC Cancer 2018;18(1):48.
15. Pallud J, Varlet P, Devaux B, et al. Diffuse low-grade oligodendrogliomas extend beyond MRI-defined abnormalities. Neurology 2010;74(21):1724–31.
16. Yordanova YN, Moritz-Gasser S, Duffau H. Awake surgery for WHO grade II gliomas within "noneloquent" areas in the left dominant hemisphere: toward a "supratotal" resection. Clinical article. J Neurosurg 2011;115(2):232–9.
17. Duffau H. Long-term outcomes after supratotal resection of diffuse low-grade gliomas: a

consecutive series with 11-year follow-up. Acta Neurochir (Wien) 2016;158(1):51–8.

18. Kawaguchi T, Sonoda Y, Shibahara I, et al. Impact of gross total resection in patients with WHO grade III glioma harboring the IDH 1/2 mutation without the 1p/19q co-deletion. J Neurooncol 2016;129(3):505–14.

19. Wijnenga MMJ, French PJ, Dubbink HJ, et al. The impact of surgery in molecularly defined low-grade glioma: an integrated clinical, radiological, and molecular analysis. Neuro Oncol 2018;20(1):103–12.

20. Chang EF, Potts MB, Keles GE, et al. Seizure characteristics and control following resection in 332 patients with low-grade gliomas. J Neurosurg 2008;108(2):227–35.

21. Ius T, Pauletto G, Isola M, et al. Surgery for insular low-grade glioma: predictors of postoperative seizure outcome. J Neurosurg 2014;120(1):12–23.

22. Barzilai O, Ben Moshe S, Sitt R, et al. Improvement in cognitive function after surgery for low-grade glioma. J Neurosurg 2018;23:1–9.

23. Johannessen TA, Mukherjee J, Viswanath P, et al. Rapid conversion of mutant IDH1 from driver to passenger in a model of human gliomagenesis. Mol Cancer Res 2016;14(10):976–83.

24. Sulkowski PL, Corso CD, Robinson ND, et al. 2-Hydroxyglutarate produced by neomorphic IDH mutations suppresses homologous recombination and induces PARP inhibitor sensitivity. Sci Transl Med 2017;9(375) [pii:eaal2463].

25. Turcan S, Fabius AW, Borodovsky A, et al. Efficient induction of differentiation and growth inhibition in IDH1 mutant glioma cells by the DNMT Inhibitor Decitabine. Oncotarget 2013;4(10):1729–36.

26. Schumacher T, Bunse L, Pusch S, et al. A vaccine targeting mutant IDH1 induces antitumour immunity. Nature 2014;512(7514):324–7.

27. Buckner JC, Shaw EG, Pugh SL, et al. Radiation plus Procarbazine, CCNU, and Vincristine in Low-Grade Glioma. N Engl J Med 2016;374(14):1344–55.

Chemotherapy Treatment and Trials in Low-Grade Gliomas

Laura E. Donovan, MD[a], Andrew B. Lassman, MS, MD[b],*

KEYWORDS

- Low-grade gliomas • Oligodendrogliomas • Astrocytomas • PCV • IDH mutations • Clinical trials
- Temozolomide

KEY POINTS

- Low-grade gliomas are molecularly and clinically heterogeneous and require an individualized approach to treatment.
- Clinical trials in low-grade gliomas are challenging because they are rare and survival data often take years to mature.
- For patients with "high-risk" low-grade gliomas, the addition of procarbazine, lomustine, and vincristine (PCV) chemotherapy to radiotherapy is associated with improved overall survival.
- Trials with molecularly target agents such as mutant IDH inhibitors are of interest, but whether they are associated with a survival benefit has yet to be determined.

INTRODUCTION

Gliomas are the most common primary brain tumors in adults.[1] Treatment varies depending on the histologic and molecular subtype and grade of the tumor as well as clinical factors such as patient characteristics and surgical accessibility of the tumor. Here we discuss the approach to adjuvant treatment in patients with diffusely infiltrating low-grade gliomas.

CLASSIFICATION AND GRADING

The World Health Organization (WHO) classifies gliomas based on presumptive cells of origin. The vast majority presumedly arise from an astrocytic lineage (astrocytomas) or, less commonly, oligodendroglial cells (oligodendrogliomas). Rarer subtypes also exist.[2]

WHO grade (I–IV) is prognostic. Grade I gliomas, such as juvenile pilocytic astrocyomas, are often curable by resection and occur in the pediatric population. Grades II through IV gliomas are diffusely infiltrating tumors that cannot be completely resected at the microscopic level and to date remain incurable. WHO grades I and II tumors are both considered "low-grade", although we focus on the grade II tumors under the definition of diffuse low-grade gliomas in this review, because they are the most common varieties in adults. Patients with such low-grade gliomas, particularly oligodendrogliamas with favorable biomarkers, may survive years or even decades after diagnosis. Therefore, treatment approaches must balance both antitumor effect and late toxicities, such as neurocognitive injury from early radiotherapy.

Disclosure: See last page of article.
[a] Departments of Neurology, Columbia University Irving Medical Center, Weill Cornell Medicine, New York-Presbyterian Hospital, 710 West 168th Street, New York, NY 10032, USA; [b] Department of Neurology and Herbert Irving Cancer Comprehensive Cancer Center, Columbia University Irving Medical Center, NewYork-Presbyterian Hospital, 710 West 168th Street, New York, NY 10032, USA
* Corresponding author.
E-mail address: ABL7@cumc.columbia.edu

In the most recent version of the WHO classification, molecular markers, specifically mutations in the *isocitrate dehydrogenase 1* (*IDH1*) and *IDH2* genes and loss of heterozygosity of chromosome arms 1p and 19q (1p/19q codeletion), play a central role in the classification of gliomas. For example, 1p/19q codeletion occurs exclusively in the context of *IDH* mutation. Both *IDH* mutation and 1p/19q codeletion are now required for a diagnosis of oligodendroglioma.[2]

The presence of an *IDH* mutation in gliomas is associated with a more indolent form of disease, a significantly longer overall survival, and is seen in up to 80% of low-grade gliomas.[3,4] In light of this finding, some groups now consider both WHO grades II and III *IDH*-mutant tumors "lower" if not "low" grade gliomas.[5]

The best approach to treatment for lower grade gliomas remains a matter of debate in the field. Clinical trials for low-grade gliomas are challenging because these tumors are rare with a relatively long median survival, and the definition of "high-risk" patients varies among trials. While trials accrue and mature, advances in the understanding of molecular biology, shifts in tumor classification, and changes in treatment patterns can present challenges for directly applying results to a contemporary population.[6,7]

RISK FACTORS FOR MORE RAPID GROWTH

Because outcomes depend on both host (age, symptoms) and tumor (size, biomarkers) factors, the questions of whom to treat, when, and with what are areas of intense interest.[8] For example, Pignatti and colleagues[9] published a set of clinical criteria to better identify patients with poorer outcomed, called "high-risk" low-grade gliomas. Factors including age greater than or equal to 40 years at diagnosis (which correlates with *IDH* wild type in tumor DNA), astrocytic rather than oligodendroglial histology (likely a surrogate for lack of 1p/19q codeletion in the current era), a preoperative maximum diameter of 6 cm, tumor crossing the midline, or the presence of neurologic deficits before surgery were all associated with worse outcome. Patients with 3 or more of these 5 "risk" factors constituted a high-risk subgroup with shorter overall survival compared with those with 0–2 risk factors.

These criteria were developed from patients participating in 2 large studies of radiotherapy conducted by the European Organization for Research and Treatment of Cancer (EORTC).[10,11] Further investigation with an independent cohort confirmed these criteria with the low-risk group having statistically significant improvements in overall (10.9 years vs 3.9 years; *P*<.0001) and progression-free survival (6.2 years vs 1.9 years; *P*<.0001) and suggested that histologic subset histology and tumor size were the primary drivers of risk.[12] Other clinical factors including Mini-Mental Status score and extent of resection were also found to be independently prognostic.[12,13] More recent studies have confirmed the importance of tumor biomarkers, including *IDH* mutation, 1p/19q codeletion, and O^6-methylguanine-DNA-methyltransferase (*MGMT*) promoter methylation status on overall survival and further research in this area is ongoing.[14–18]

However, the definition of risk in clinical trials remains variable. The Radiation Therapy Oncology Group (RTOG) trial 9802 defined high risk low-grade gliomas as those occurring in patients 40 years of age or older or in those less than 40 years of age who underwent less than gross-total resection.[19] EORTC 22033-26033, by contrast, defined high-risk patients as those with at least 1 of the following characteristics: age 40 years or older, progressive disease, tumor size greater than 5 cm, tumor crossing the midline, or neurologic symptoms.[20] RTOG 0424 required patients to have at least 3 risk factors for recurrence (age ≥40, tumor size ≥6 cm, tumor crossing the midline, astrocytic histology, or preoperative neurologic deficits).[21] Therefore, cross-trial comparisons of outcomes are difficult.

TREATMENT OF LOW-RISK DISEASE

When radiotherapy is administered, the required dose is lower (approximately 50 Gy) than the dose used for high-grade tumors (approximately 60 Gy) without compromising survival and with less toxicity.[10,22] However, EORTC 22485 reported survival of approximately 7.3 years regardless of whether radiotherapy was administered at diagnosis or progression.[11] Therefore, delaying radiotherapy does not seem to compromise survival and deferring it may be reasonable in some patients. Similarly, recent data from EORTC demonstrated that progression-free survival after initial treatment with temozolomide (without radiotherapy) was similar to that with radiotherapy (without chemotherapy), although the results were impacted by molecular subgrouping and survival data are immature.[20]

This finding has led some investigators to favor temozolomide as an initial strategy with deferred radiotherapy. However, temozolomide also can induce changes in the molecular profile of the tumor. In support of observation, there is some evidence suggesting that early treatment of low-grade gliomas with temozolomide may lead to a hypermutated genotype. In a comparison of low-grade gliomas at initial diagnosis and at recurrence, 6 of 10 tumors treated with temozolomide were found to have a hypermutated genotype with driver mutations activating the retinoblastoma (RB) and mammalian target of rapamycin (mTOR) pathways, suggesting that temozolomide-induced mutagenesis can contribute to transformation of low-grade tumors into high-grade tumors through the inactivation of mismatch repair pathway genes.[23,24] Whether this phenomenon is clinically significant remains to be seen.

Of note, EORTC 22485 demonstrated that delayed radiotherapy did not negatively influence survival relative to observation, but that trial did not test radiochemotherapy, that is, radiotherapy combined either with temozolomide or with procarbazine, lomustine (CCNU), and vincristine (together, PCV). Therefore, it is possible that, although deferring radiotherapy does not shorten survival, deferring both may. This finding is of particular concern in the context of long-term results from RTOG 9802 (discussed elsewhere in this article), demonstrating that adding chemotherapy (with PCV) to radiotherapy prolongs survival. As a corollary, EORTC 22033-26033 showed that temozolomide alone at best is associated with similar survival to radiotherapy alone.[20] In more detail, this phase III trial randomized 477 low-grade glioma patients with at least 1 high-risk feature to either temozolomide or radiotherapy.[20] Preliminary results suggest no difference in the median progression-free survival between the 2 groups (39 months with temozolomide vs 46 months with radiotherapy; $P = .22$).[20] Follow-up is ongoing and we await both further molecular correlations and mature survival analyses.[20]

By extrapolation, temozolomide alone is likely to be inferior to combined radiochemotherapy. Therefore, if treatment is administered, either chemotherapy or radiotherapy alone are likely associated with shortened survival relative to radiochemotherapy.

In addition, it is clear that not all clinically defined low-risk low-grade gliomas behave as such. In 1998, the RTOG initiated a phase II observational study of patients with low-risk low-grade gliomas, defined as age less than 40 years without residual disease after resection (neurosurgeon defined). These patients were observed without further adjuvant treatment and the 2- and 5-year overall survival rates were 99% and 93%, respectively; however, more than 50% had obvious tumor growth within 5 years, a rate much higher than anticipated. Further analysis found preoperative tumor size (≥4 cm), astrocytic histology, and

evidence of residual disease greater than 1 cm on brain imaging were all predictive of shorter progression-free survival.[25]

However, upfront treatment has consequences in patients who survive 5 or more years. Therefore, deferring treatment entirely may be appropriate in those with low-risk disease: patients less than 40 years of age with less than 1 cm of residual disease on post-operative MRI, and a favorable histologic and molecular profiles, specifically WHO grade II oligodendrogliomas (IDH mutant, 1p/19q codeleted). For example, in RTOG 9802, patients with oligodendrogliomas had a median survival of more than 13.3 years (median not reached) with combination radiotherapy + PCV and 10.8 years with radiotherapy alone.[19] The risk of neurocognitive injury from radiotherapy in this time frame is not trivial and neurocognitive decline has been demonstrated to have a negative impact on quality of life.[26,27] Neurocognitive results from RTOG 9802 are still pending. Although the short-term follow-up (5–6 years) has shown an improvement in cognitive function with decreased tumor burden after radiotherapy,[28] very late follow-up studies (>12 years) demonstrate deficits in attention, information processing, and executive function in patients with low-grade glioma who received early radiotherapy compared with those who delayed radiotherapy.[29]

Accordingly, in these patients at the lowest risk, observation alone or upfront chemotherapy with delayed radiotherapy at the time of progression may be reasonable approaches to avoid late neurotoxicity from early radiotherapy, recognizing that alkylator therapy may have its own consequences. Deferred radiotherapy was assessed in a small North Central Cancer Treatment Group/Mayo Clinic trial evaluating 28 patients with low-grade oligodendrogliomas undergoing subtotal resection. Patients were treated upfront with an intensified PCV regimen[30] with radiotherapy given at progression. Of 25 evaluable patients, blinded radiology review demonstrated a decrease in tumor size with PCV alone in 52% of cases.[31]

Subsequently, RTOG 9402 and EORTC 96951, 2 large, phase III, randomized, controlled trials assessing radiotherapy with or without PCV in anaplastic oligodendrogliomas demonstrated similar results for the subset of patients with molecularly defined oligodendrogliomas (1p/19q codeleted, IDH mutant), regardless of whether PCV was administered before or after radiotherapy.[32,33] Based on these results, it may be reasonable to defer RT to progression, although whether or not a significant delay to radiotherapy after PCV has an impact on overall survival remains unknown.

TREATMENT OF HIGH-RISK DISEASE

Patients with high-risk low-grade gliomas derive a clear benefit from adjuvant treatment after resection. Currently, the strongest evidence for treatment comes from RTOG 9802. This phase III randomized, controlled trial compared radiotherapy to radiotherapy followed by PCV. Although the preliminary results demonstrated an improvement in progression-free survival but not overall survival with the addition of PCV to radiotherapy,[34] long-term follow-up revealed a clear benefit of chemoradiotherapy with nearly doubled overall survival (13.3 years vs 7.8 years; P = .003).[19] Subgroup analysis revealed that this benefit was most pronounced in patients with oligodendrogliomas and oligoastrocytomas, but even patients with astrocytomas benefited. Patients with *IDH*-mutated tumors also seemed to derive greater benefit from combination therapy compared with those with *IDH* wild-type tumors, although these results must be interpreted with caution given the small numbers in subgroup analyses. Based on the results of this trial, radiotherapy alone for adjuvant treatment of high risk low-grade gliomas is now considered inadequate.[19]

PCV OR TEMOZOLOMIDE

Whether PCV is the appropriate adjuvant chemotherapy regimen for all low-grade gliomas remains a matter of debate. While RTOG 9802 was continuing to accrue and mature, temozolomide, an oral alkylating agent designed to penetrate the blood–brain barrier, became widely accepted as the chemotherapy of choice for gliomas of all grades and histologies after the results of the landmark EORTC 22981/26981 and NCIC CE.3 trial demonstrating an overall survival benefit with the addition of concurrent and adjuvant temozolomide to radiotherapy vs. radiotherapy alone in patients with newly diagnosed glioblastoma.[35] Temozolomide is reasonably well-tolerated; only 16% of patients experienced grade III or IV adverse hematologic effects and less than 5% discontinued for toxicity in the glioblastoma trial.[35]

Conversely, PCV[36] is not a trivial regimen to administer and adverse effects are common. PCV is typically administered over 8 weeks and consists of lomsutine (CCNU) dosed at 110 mg/m^2 on day 1 followed procarbazine 60 mg/m^2 per day on days 8 to 21, both oral drugs taken at home. Procarbazine is manufactured only in 50-mg tablets, which requires the total dose to be rounded and divided over 14 days. Patients must travel to an infusion center on days 8 and 29 to receive intravenous vincristine at 1.4 mg/m^2 (with a 2-mg cap). In many cases, neuropathy prevents administration of the second vincristine dose[30] and myelosuppression necessitates dose reductions of procarbazine and CCNU in subsequent cycles. For example, in RTOG 9802, blood or bone marrow toxicities were seen in the majority of patients, with 64% experiencing grade III or IV toxicities. Nausea, vomiting, fatigue, and weight loss were also common and occasionally severe.[19] On average, patients completed only 3 to 4 of the recommended 6 cycles,[19] similar to other trials of PCV in patients with anaplastic gliomas.[32,33]

For 1p/19q codeleted anaplastic oligodendrogliomas, there is increasing evidence to suggest that PCV may be more effective than temozolomide, including randomized data,[37] as reviewed elsewhere,[38,39] although this outcome is not universally accepted. Perhaps it is not surprising that the addition of PCV to radiotherapy would result in a survival benefit in patients with oligodendrogliomas in RTOG 9802 because oligodendrogliomas are more chemosensitive than their astrocytic counterparts, in part because of the presence of 1p/19q codeletion. Whether the potential for superior efficacy of PCV over temozolomide justifies the added toxicity is unclear and is particularly unclear for low-grade astrocytomas that, by definition, do not harbor the 1p/19q codeletion and are less chemosensitive.

However, anaplastic gliomas without 1p/19q codeletion but with *IDH* mutation also seem to benefit from PCV, although the magnitude is less than in codeleted tumors.[40] *IDH* mutation is much more common in low-grade astrocytomas compared with anaplastic astrocytomas.[4] Therefore, patients with low-grade astrocytomas still derive some benefit from chemotherapy, as observed in RTOG 9802,[19] although temozolomide may be more appropriate in this population given the toxicities associated with PCV.

RTOG 0424 provides some data in support of temozolomide. This single arm phase II study evaluated radiotherapy with concurrent temozolomide followed by adjuvant temozolomide in patients with low-grade glioma and at least 3 high-risk features. Preliminary results suggest an improvement in overall survival at 3 years compared with historical controls treated with radiotherapy alone (73.1% vs 54.0%; P<.001); however, the data are still maturing as the median overall survival has not yet been reached.[21] Given this is a single-arm study without a control group, final results should also be interpreted with caution.

INVESTIGATIONAL AGENTS

Radiotherapy, PCV, and temozolomide are antiquated approaches to the treatment of these diseases; newer, "targeted" agents, such as mutant IDH inhibitors, are intriguing. *IDH* mutations occur very early in tumorigenesis and the resultant buildup of the oncometabolite 2-hydroxyglutarate leads to a variety of alterations in histone and DNA methylation that drive the development of gliomas and other tumors.[41] The US Food and Drug Administration recently approved enasidenib, a mutant IDH2 inhibitor, for the treatment of relapsed or refractory acute myelogenous leukemia.[42] Inhibitors of mutant IDH1 and IDH2 are of interest in low-grade gliomas as well, and clinical trials are ongoing. These trials are subject to the same challenges as other trials in low-grade gliomas, namely, that accrual occurs slowly and it takes many for survival results to mature.[43] Although the overall survival benefit remains unknown, and trials today have not shown objective responses (defined typically as a $\geq$50% decrease in cross-sectional area on MRI), there is preliminary evidence to suggest these drugs may slow the growth rate for *IDH*-mutant tumors, which could have a clinically meaningful impact on outcome. Additional studies are ongoing.[44,45]

There is also evidence to suggest that *IDH* mutation may induce a BRCA-like phenotype with defects in homologous recombination. These defects may confer sensitivity to poly(adenosine 5'-diphosphate-ribose) inhibitors and clinical trials are currently underway for these agents as well.[46]

SUMMARY

The treatment of low-grade gliomas remains challenging in part because of molecular and clinical heterogeneity. In patients with high-risk clinical or molecular features, adjuvant treatment after resection should be pursued. Based on the results of RTOG 9802, the addition of adjuvant PCV chemotherapy to radiotherapy prolongs survival vs. radiotherapy alone, particularly for oligodendrogliomas. Trials with temozolomide preliminarily show some benefit as well. Although PCV may be the best option for patients with molecularly defined oligodendrogliomas, temozolomide may be effective in low-grade astrocytomas with less toxicity, although final analyses and molecular data are pending. In low-risk patients with a median survival of a decade or more, the potential benefit of adjuvant therapy must be weighed against the risk for long-term side effects. In these patients, chemotherapy alone or observation may be reasonable. Ongoing trials with molecularly targeted therapies are of interest, but their impact remains to be determined.

DISCLOSURE

Within the last year, A.B. Lassman has received personal compensation (consulting fees/honoraria) from GLG, NCI, Guidepoint Global, Sapience Therapeutics, Olson Research Group, Bioclinica, Focus Forward Incentives, WebMD, Health Advisors Bureau/Medefield, Celgene, ASCO, prIME Oncology, RICCA Group, Agios, and several law firms as a medical expert; travel support from Abbvie, Aios, Celgene, Novocure, NRG Oncology Foundation, and Tocagen; and research support (to the institution) from AbbVie, Novartis, Karyopharm, Genentech/Roche, Novocure, Aeterna Zentaris, Pfizer, Bayer/Onyx, Agenus, GSK, Stemline Therapeutics, Northwest Biotherapeutics, Plexxikon, Tocagen, Regeneron, VBL Therapeutics, e-Therapeutics, BMS, ImmunoCellular Therapeutics, Merck, Amgen, Celldex, Millennium, MedImmune, Boehringer Ingelheim, Kadmon, RTOG Foundation, Boston Biomedical, BeiGene, Diffusion Pharmaceuticals, Agios, Celgene, Vascular Biogenics, Angiochem, DC Vax, and Orbus. L.E. Donovan has nothing to disclose. The work was conducted with the support of the William Rhodes and Louise Tilzer-Rhodes Center for Glioblastoma at NewYork-Presbyterian Hospital.

REFERENCES

1. Ostrom QT, Gittleman H, Liao P, et al. CBTRUS statistical report: primary brain and other central nervous system tumors diagnosed in the United States in 2010-2014. Neuro Oncol 2017;19(suppl_5):v1–88.

2. Louis DN, Perry A, Reifenberger G, et al. The 2016 World Health Organization classification of tumors of the central nervous system: a summary. Acta Neuropathol 2016;131(6):803–20.

3. Parsons DW, Jones S, Zhang X, et al. An integrated genomic analysis of human glioblastoma multiforme. Science 2008;321(5897):1807–12.

4. Yan H, Parsons DW, Jin G, et al. IDH1 and IDH2 mutations in gliomas. N Engl J Med 2009;360(8):765–73.

5. Cancer Genome Atlas Research N, Brat DJ, Verhaak RG, et al. Comprehensive, integrative genomic analysis of diffuse lower-grade gliomas. N Engl J Med 2015;372(26):2481–98.

6. Panageas KS, Iwamoto FM, Cloughesy TF, et al. Initial treatment patterns over time for anaplastic oligodendroglial tumors. Neuro Oncol 2012;14(6):761–7.

7. van den Bent MJ. Chemotherapy for low-grade glioma: when, for whom, which regimen? Curr Opin Neurol 2015;28(6):633–938.

8. Schaff LR, Lassman AB. Indications for treatment: is observation or chemotherapy alone a reasonable approach in the management of low-grade gliomas? Semin Radiat Oncol 2015;25(3):203–9.

9. Pignatti F, van den Bent M, Curran D, et al. Prognostic factors for survival in adult patients with cerebral low-grade glioma. J Clin Oncol 2002;20(8): 2076–84.

10. Karim AB, Maat B, Hatlevoll R, et al. A randomized trial on dose-response in radiation therapy of low-grade cerebral glioma: European Organization for Research and Treatment of Cancer (EORTC) Study 22844. Int J Radiat Oncol Biol Phys 1996;36(3): 549–56.

11. van den Bent MJ, Afra D, de Witte O, et al. Long-term efficacy of early versus delayed radiotherapy for low-grade astrocytoma and oligodendroglioma in adults: the EORTC 22845 randomised trial. Lancet 2005;366(9490):985–90.

12. Daniels TB, Brown PD, Felten SJ, et al. Validation of EORTC prognostic factors for adults with low-grade glioma: a report using intergroup 86-72-51. Int J Radiat Oncol Biol Phys 2011;81(1):218–24.

13. Smith JS, Chang EF, Lamborn KR, et al. Role of extent of resection in the long-term outcome of low-grade hemispheric gliomas. J Clin Oncol 2008; 26(8):1338–45.

14. Wijnenga MMJ, Dubbink HJ, French PJ, et al. Molecular and clinical heterogeneity of adult diffuse low-grade IDH wild-type gliomas: assessment of TERT promoter mutation and chromosome 7 and 10 copy number status allows superior prognostic stratification. Acta Neuropathol 2017;134(6):957–9.

15. Aibaidula A, Chan AK, Shi Z, et al. Adult IDH wild-type lower-grade gliomas should be further stratified. Neuro Oncol 2017;19(10):1327–37.

16. Chan AK, Yao Y, Zhang Z, et al. Combination genetic signature stratifies lower-grade gliomas better than histological grade. Oncotarget 2015;6(25):20885–901.

17. Everhard SS, Kaloshi GG, Crinière EE, et al. MGMT methylation: a marker of response to temozolomide in low-grade gliomas. Ann Neurol 2006;60(6): 740–3.

18. Bell EH, Zhang P, Fisher BJ, et al. Association of MGMT promoter methylation status with survival outcomes in patients with high-risk glioma treated with radiotherapy and temozolomide: an analysis from the NRG Oncology/RTOG 0424 trial. JAMA Oncol 2018;4(10):1405–9.

19. Buckner JC, Shaw EG, Pugh SL, et al. Radiation plus procarbazine, CCNU, and vincristine in low-grade glioma. N Engl J Med 2016;374(14):1344–55.

20. Baumert BG, Hegi ME, van den Bent MJ, et al. Temozolomide chemotherapy versus radiotherapy in high-risk low-grade glioma (EORTC 22033-26033): a randomised, open-label, phase 3 intergroup study. Lancet Oncol 2016;17(11):1521–32.

21. Fisher BJ, Hu C, Macdonald DR, et al. Phase 2 study of temozolomide-based chemoradiation therapy for high-risk low-grade gliomas: preliminary results of Radiation Therapy Oncology Group 0424. Int J Radiat Oncol Biol Phys 2015;91(3): 497–504.

22. Shaw E, Arusell R, Scheithauer B, et al. Prospective randomized trial of low- versus high-dose radiation therapy in adults with supratentorial low-grade glioma: initial report of a North Central Cancer Treatment Group/Radiation Therapy Oncology Group/Eastern Cooperative Oncology Group study. J Clin Oncol 2002;20(9):2267–76.

23. van Thuijl HF, Mazor T, Johnson BE, et al. Evolution of DNA repair defects during malignant progression of low-grade gliomas after temozolomide treatment. Acta Neuropathol 2015;129(4):597–607.

24. Johnson BE, Mazor T, Hong C, et al. Mutational analysis reveals the origin and therapy-driven evolution of recurrent glioma. Science 2014;343(6167): 189–93.

25. Shaw EG, Berkey B, Coons SW, et al. Recurrence following neurosurgeon-determined gross-total resection of adult supratentorial low-grade glioma: results of a prospective clinical trial. J Neurosurg 2008;109(5):835–41.

26. Li J, Bentzen SM, Li J, et al. Relationship between neurocognitive function and quality of life after whole-brain radiotherapy in patients with brain metastasis. Int J Radiat Oncol Biol Phys 2008; 71(1):64–70.

27. Lieberman AN, Foo SH, Ransohoff J, et al. Long term survival among patients with malignant brain tumors. Neurosurgery 1982;10(4):450–3.

28. Prabhu RS, Won M, Shaw EG, et al. Effect of the addition of chemotherapy to radiotherapy on cognitive function in patients with low-grade glioma: secondary analysis of RTOG 98-02. J Clin Oncol 2014; 32(6):535–41.

29. Douw L, Klein M, Fagel SS, et al. Cognitive and radiological effects of radiotherapy in patients with low-grade glioma: long-term follow-up. Lancet Neurol 2009;8(9):810–8.

30. Cairncross G, Macdonald D, Ludwin S, et al. Chemotherapy for anaplastic oligodendroglioma. National Cancer Institute of Canada Clinical Trials Group. J Clin Oncol 1994;12(10):2013–21.

31. Buckner JC, Gesme D Jr, O'Fallon JR, et al. Phase II trial of procarbazine, lomustine, and vincristine as initial therapy for patients with low-grade oligodendroglioma or oligoastrocytoma: efficacy and associations with chromosomal abnormalities. J Clin Oncol 2003;21(2):251–5.

32. van den Bent MJ, Brandes AA, Taphoorn MJ, et al. Adjuvant procarbazine, lomustine, and vincristine chemotherapy in newly diagnosed anaplastic oligodendroglioma: long-term follow-up of EORTC brain

tumor group study 26951. J Clin Oncol 2013;31(3): 344–50.

33. Cairncross G, Wang M, Shaw E, et al. Phase III trial of chemoradiotherapy for anaplastic oligodendroglioma: long-term results of RTOG 9402. J Clin Oncol 2013;31(3):337–43.

34. Shaw EG, Wang M, Coons SW, et al. Randomized trial of radiation therapy plus procarbazine, lomustine, and vincristine chemotherapy for supratentorial adult low-grade glioma: initial results of RTOG 9802. J Clin Oncol 2012;30(25):3065–70.

35. Stupp R, Mason WP, van den Bent MJ, et al. Radiotherapy plus concomitant and adjuvant temozolomide for glioblastoma. N Engl J Med 2005;352(10): 987–96.

36. Levin VA, Edwards MS, Wright DC, et al. Modified procarbazine, CCNU, and vincristine (PCV 3) combination chemotherapy in the treatment of malignant brain tumors. Cancer Treat Rep 1980;64(2–3): 237–44.

37. Wick W, Roth P, Hartmann C, et al. Long-term analysis of the NOA-04 randomized phase III trial of sequential radiochemotherapy of anaplastic glioma with PCV or temozolomide. Neuro Oncol 2016; 18(11):1529–37.

38. Lassman AB. Procarbazine, lomustine and vincristine or temozolomide: which is the better regimen? CNS Oncol 2015;4(5):341–6.

39. Lassman AB, Cloughesy TF. Biomarkers in NOA-04: another piece to the puzzle. Neuro Oncol 2016; 18(11):1467–9.

40. Cairncross JG, Wang M, Jenkins RB, et al. Benefit from procarbazine, lomustine, and vincristine in oligodendroglial tumors is associated with mutation of IDH. J Clin Oncol 2014;32(8): 783–90.

41. Waitkus MS, Diplas BH, Yan H. Biological role and therapeutic potential of IDH mutations in cancer. Cancer Cell 2018;34(2):186–95.

42. Nassereddine S, Lap CJ, Haroun F, et al. The role of mutant IDH1 and IDH2 inhibitors in the treatment of acute myeloid leukemia. Ann Hematol 2017;96(12): 1983–91.

43. van den Bent MJ, Jaeckle K, Baumert B, et al. RTOG 9802: good wines need aging. J Clin Oncol 2013; 31(5):653–4.

44. Mellinghoff IK, Tauat M, Maher E, et al. ACTR-46 AG-120, a first-in-class mutant IDH1 inhibitor in patients with recurrent or progressive IDH1 mutant glioma: updated results from the phase 1 non-enhancing glioma population. Neuro Oncol 2017; 19(Suppl 6). e10–11.

45. Mellinghoff IK, Penas-Prado M, Peters KB, et al. Phase 1 study of AG-881, an inhibitor of mutant IDH1/IDH2, in patients with advanced IDH-mutant solid tumors, including glioma. J Clin Oncol 2018; 36(Suppl) [abstract: 2002].

46. Sulkowski PL, Corso CD, Robinson ND, et al. 2-Hydroxyglutarate produced by neomorphic IDH mutations suppresses homologous recombination and induces PARP inhibitor sensitivity. Sci Transl Med 2017;9(375) [pii:eaal2463].

Low-Grade Glioma Radiotherapy Treatment and Trials

Tony J.C. Wang, MD[a,b], Minesh P. Mehta, MD[c,*]

KEYWORDS

- Low-grade glioma • Radiotherapy • Trials

KEY POINTS

- Low-grade gliomas represent an uncommon but important class of primary brain tumors, especially because of long survivorship.
- Radiotherapy is one of the main components of treatment for patients with low-grade glioma and is associated with increased progression-free survival and improved overall survival as part of combined modality therapy.
- Optimal timing of radiotherapy for low-grade glioma has historically remained controversial owing to concerns of potential side effects and malignant transformation, but recent data point to early use of radiotherapy with the exception of patients with very low-risk, low-grade gliomas.
- Recent molecular evaluation has led to incorporating molecular markers in grading and risk categorization.
- Ongoing trials for low-grade gliomas seem to be promising toward furthering our understanding of these tumors and potentially prolonging progression-free and overall survival.

INTRODUCTION

Low-grade gliomas are slow-growing World Health Organization (WHO) grade I or II primary brain tumors that predominantly affect young adults. WHO grade II tumors present most commonly during the fourth decade of life.[1] Low-grade gliomas are composed of various distinct tumors based on histopathology. For this review, WHO grade II low-grade gliomas are generally separated into 2 categories: diffuse astrocytoma and oligodendroglioma. In 2016, the WHO reclassified low-grade glioma by combining classic histopathologic features with key molecular markers, including isocitrate dehydrogenase (IDH) mutation and 1p/19q codeletion status, reflecting the fact that prognosis is more strongly associated with molecular diagnostic features.[2] Unlike their more common high-grade glioma counterparts, patients with low-grade glioma have a more favorable prognosis. The treatment

Funding: None.

Conflict of Interest: Dr T.J.C. Wang reports personal fees and nonfinancial support from AbbVie, nonfinancial support from Merck, personal fees from AstraZeneca, personal fees from Doximity, nonfinancial support from Novocure, personal fees and nonfinancial support from Elekta, and personal fees from Wolters Kluwer, outside the submitted work. Dr M.P. Mehta reports consulting fees from Abbvie, Celgene, Tocagen; DSMB for Monteris; and stock options from Oncoceutics for being on the Board of Directors.

[a] Department of Radiation Oncology, Columbia University Medical Center, 622 West 168th Street, BNH B-11, New York, NY 10032, USA; [b] Herbert Irving Comprehensive Cancer Center, Columbia University Medical Center, 630 West 168th Street, New York, NY 10032, USA; [c] Miami Cancer Institute, Baptist Hospital, 8900 North Kendall Drive, Miami, FL 33176, USA

* Corresponding author.

E-mail address: MineshM@baptisthealth.net

Neurosurg Clin N Am 30 (2019) 111–118

https://doi.org/10.1016/j.nec.2018.08.008

paradigm for low-grade glioma typically consists of surgery, observation, chemotherapy, and/or radiation therapy (RT). Owing to longer survival outcomes compared with high-grade gliomas, treatment decisions regarding observation versus aggressive intervention must take into account potential acute and long-term side effects that may impact quality of life. Recent clinical trials and RT technological advances have broadened our understanding and impacted the diagnosis and treatment of low-grade gliomas. In this review, we provide an update on the role of RT for low-grade glioma, specifically regarding WHO grade II tumors. We also discuss advances in radiation technology, as well as recent and ongoing clinical trials related to RT for low-grade glioma.

PROGNOSIS: UNDERSTANDING WHO TO TREAT

WHO grade II low-grade gliomas encompass a variety of tumors with different behaviors and prognoses. Patients with higher risk features for tumor progression are presumed to receive the greatest benefit from therapeutic intervention, but of course this specific hypothesis has not been tested. In 2002, Pignatti and colleagues[3] performed a multivariate analysis from the EORTC 22844 and 22845 trials reporting 5 unfavorable prognostic factors for survival: age 40 years or older, astrocytoma histology subtype, maximum diameter of 6 cm or greater, tumor crossing midline, and the presence of neurologic deficits before surgery. Low-risk patients, defined by the presence of up to 2 risk factors, displayed a median survival of 7.7 years versus 3.2 years among high-risk patients having 3 or more risk factors. More recently, secondary analyses from clinical trials have identified important genetic mutations that are more prognostic than histopathology, including mutations in *IDH*, *ATRX*, and *TERT* promoters, and combined chromosomal deletions of 1p and 19q.[4–7] The presence of mutations in either *IDH* 1 or 2 is associated with significantly longer overall survival, leading the 2016 WHO classification to use this as a key variable.[8,9] In RTOG 9802, a phase III trial for adult high-risk low-grade gliomas (here defined as patients <40 years old with an incomplete resection or >40 years old with any extent of resection), patients were randomized to RT alone versus RT plus 6 cycles of procarbazine, lomustine, and vincristine (PCV) chemotherapy. Compared with median survival of 7.8 years with RT and 13.3 years with CRT among all enrolled patients, IDH-mutated patients displayed a median survival of 10.1 years with RT, whereas the median

survival with chemoradiotherapy (CRT) was not reached. Combined chromosomal 1p and 19q codeletion as well as 1;19 translocation are also associated with superior overall and progression-free survival in low-grade glioma.[6] In a secondary analysis of the NCCTG/RTOG/ECOG trial,[10] a randomized trial for patients with low-grade glioma comparing 50.4 Gy versus 64.8 Gy, Jenkins and colleagues[6] reported a median survival of 11.9 years for patients with 1;19 translocation versus 8.1 years without this alteration. Specifically for oligodendroglioma, the median survival was 13.0 years for patients with a 1;19 translocation versus 9.1 years without it. The use of molecular biomarkers beyond IDH and 1p19q deletion status as potential predictive factors for RT sensitivity holds significant promise toward improving individualized treatment decision making.

THE ROLE OF RADIOTHERAPY FOR LOW-GRADE GLIOMAS

The goals of RT for low-grade glioma are to improve tumor control and survival while preventing/delaying malignant transformation and limiting the acute and late effects of treatment that may degrade quality of life. Thus, understanding current data on RT for low-grade glioma is critical for informing treatment decisions. Multiple randomized, clinical trials have been published examining the roles of and dosing for RT in low-grade glioma (**Table 1**). The NCCTG/RTOG/ECOG trial randomized 203 adult patients with low-grade glioma to 50.4 Gy versus 64.8 Gy.[10] No statistically significant 5-year overall survival difference was observed between the 50.4-Gy and 64.8-Gy arms (64% vs 72%, respectively). The 5-year progression-free survival was also not statistically different between arms (55% in the 50.4-Gy arm vs 52% in the 64.8-Gy arm, respectively). Notably, a secondary analysis on the cognitive effects of RT using the Mini-Mental State Examination found that only 5.3% of patients deteriorated by 5 years, although most patients with low-grade glioma maintained stable neurocognitive function.[11] Another randomized trial studying radiotherapy dose for low-grade glioma was the EORTC 22844 study, which randomized 343 patients to 45 Gy versus 59.4 Gy.[12] The 5-year overall survival rates were 58% in the 45-Gy arm versus 59% in the 59.4-Gy arm, which was not significantly different. Similarly, the 5-year progression-free survival was not significantly different between the arms (47% for 45 Gy vs 50% for 59.4 Gy, respectively). Neither randomized trial showed an overall or progression-free survival benefit from

Table 1
Randomized trials on radiotherapy for low-grade gliomas

Trial	Treatment Arm	Number of Patients	Median Progression-Free Survival	5-y Progression-Free Survival (%)	Median Overall Survival	5-y Overall Survival (%)
EORTC 22844[12]	45 Gy in 25 fractions	171	NA	47	NA	58
	59.4 Gy in 33 fractions	172	NA	50	NA	59
EORTC 22845[13]	Observation	157	3.4 y	35	7.2 y	66
	54 Gy in 30 fractions	157	5.3 y	55	7.4 y	68
NCCTG/ RTOG/ ECOG[10]	50.4 Gy in 33 fractions	101	NA	55	NA	72
	64.8 Gy in 36 fractions	102	NA	52	NA	64
RTOG 9802[8]	54 Gy in 30 fraction	126	4.0 y	61	7.8 y	72
	54 Gy in 30 fraction plus 6 cycles PCV	125	10.4 y	44	13.3 y	63
EORTC 22033-26033[15]	12 cycles of temozolomide	237	39 mo	29	NR	NA
	50.4 Gy in 28 fractions	240	46 mo	40	NR	NA

Abbreviations: ECOG, Eastern Cooperative Oncology Group; EORTC, European Organisation for Research and Treatment of Cancer; NA, not available; NCCT, North Central Cancer Treatment Group; NR, not reached; PCV, procarbazine, lomustine, and vincristine; RTOG, Radiation Therapy Oncology Group.

dose escalation. In the United States, it is generally accepted that a reasonable RT dose for low-grade glioma is 50 to 54 Gy to balance efficacy and toxicity.

One randomized, clinical trial examined the timing of RT for low-grade glioma. The EORTC 22845 trial randomized 314 patients with low-grade glioma to early RT of 54 Gy vs deferred RT until the time of progression.[13] Median progression-free survival was 5.3 years in the early RT arm versus 3.4 years in the deferred RT arm ($P < .0001$). However, because the majority of "observed" patients (65%) received RT, median overall survival was similar between the early and deferred RT arms (7.4 years vs 7.2 years, respectively). Importantly, the proportion of patients with seizures at 1 year was significantly lower in the early RT group compared with the deferred RT group (25% vs 41%, respectively; $P = .0329$), implying that tumor control has significant clinical benefit. The authors concluded that early RT improves progression-free survival and control of seizures, but not overall survival. Quality of life was not studied and, therefore, whether shorter time to progression impacts neurocognitive deterioration is not known.

The lack of overall survival benefit has been used by some to justify deferring RT until disease progression. This strategy can be considered for patients with low-grade glioma with highly favorable prognostic features and minimal known disease (eg, those younger than 40 years of age, with MRI-confirmed gross totally resected *IDH* mutated WHO grade II oligodendroglioma), provided they are observed carefully. RTOG 9802 included an observation cohort of so-called low-risk low-grade gliomas that underwent resection without adjuvant therapy. One hundred eleven patients younger than 40 years who had achieved a surgeon-determined gross total resection were entered into the study; the overall survival rates at 2 and 5 years were 99% and 93%, respectively. The progression-free survival rates at 2 and 5 years were 82% and only 48%. Three factors predicted significantly poorer progression-free survival: (1) preoperative tumor diameter of 4 cm or greater, (2) astrocytoma/oligoastrocytoma histologic type, and (3) residual tumor 1 cm or greater according to postoperative MRI. A review of the postoperative MRI results revealed that 59% of patients had less than 1 cm of residual disease (with a subsequent 26% recurrence rate), 32% had 1 to 2 cm of residual disease (with a subsequent 68% recurrence rate), and 9% had more than 2 cm of residual disease (with a subsequent 89% recurrence rate).[14]

The recent publication of the mature results of the treatment arms for higher risk patients with low-grade glioma enrolled in the RTOG 9802 trial showed that patients with low-grade glioma selected for postoperative RT should also receive adjuvant chemotherapy. Two hundred fifty-one patients with low-grade glioma were randomized to postoperative RT with or without 6 cycles of adjuvant PCV.[8] The median progression-free survival was 4.0 years in the RT arm versus 10.4 years in the CRT arm (P < .001). The median overall survival was also significantly improved for the CRT arm versus RT arm (13.3 years vs 7.8 years, respectively). The added survival benefit from PCV was observed in all low-grade glioma histologies, with the greatest effect size in oligodendroglioma patients. Of note, there were significantly more grade III and IV hematologic toxicities in the CRT arm, although there were no treatment-related deaths.

A significant way to interpret these data is to recognize that, because RT alone has not been shown to improve overall survival, the results of that arm could be viewed as equivalent to "observation" (which in effect means delayed salvage RT); however, RT in combination with PCV produces the longest overall survival ever described in a clinical trial context and, therefore, it is fair to ask whether chemotherapy alone (with delayed RT) could produce similar results. The EORTC 22033-26033 study randomized 477 patients with low-grade glioma with at least 1 risk factor as defined by Pignatti and colleagues[3] to receive 50.4 Gy RT alone versus chemotherapy alone using 12 cycles of adjuvant dose-intense temozolomide (TMZ).[15] In their preliminary analysis, the median progression free-survival was 39 months in the TMZ arm versus 46 months in the RT arm (P = .22). Of note, patients with IDH mutation and non–1p19q-codeleted tumors had longer progression-free survival in the RT arm (55 months) versus the TMZ arm (36 months), with a hazard ratio of 1.86 (P = .0043), but there were no differences in progression-free survival for the IDH mutated, codeleted, or the IDH wild-type tumors. Mature overall survival data from this trial are still pending, but the relatively short time to progression on chemotherapy alone meant that a considerable proportion of patients on that arm rather rapidly received salvage RT, thereby likely making the overall survival interpretation possibly difficult. A separate preliminary analysis among patients with low-grade glioma of the effects of TMZ or RT on health-related quality of life and global cognitive functioning found no differences, belying the oft-quoted rationale for delaying radiotherapy, that is, the assumed cognitive and quality of life decline associated with its use, which in this randomized trial was no better or worse than TMZ

alone.[16] Although these preliminary results shed some light regarding the question of TMZ versus RT as monotherapy, overall survival and quality of life results are pending longer follow-up. In the meantime, nonrandomized data emerging from institutions where the TMZ-first principle had supplanted the upfront use of RT provide some interesting insights. Recently, Wahl and colleagues[17] presented the findings of a single-arm phase II trial on 120 patients with WHO grade II gliomas (57 oligodendrogliomas, 20 oligoastrocytomas, 43 astrocytomas) treated with TMZ first. Patients received monthly cycles of TMZ for up to 1 year or until progression and were monitored with serial MRI at baseline and every 2 months during treatment. The median progression-free survival was 4.2 years and the median overall survival was 9.7 years. The authors concluded that "patients with high-risk [low-grade glioma] receiving adjuvant TMZ (alone) demonstrated a high rate of radiographic stability and favorable survival outcomes while meaningfully delaying RT." However, the more germane question is whether this approach of sequential use of TMZ followed by delayed RT is superior to the CRT approach adopted in RTOG 9802 or not. In RTOG 9802, the median progression-free survival was 4.0 years in the RT arm (comparable with TMZ

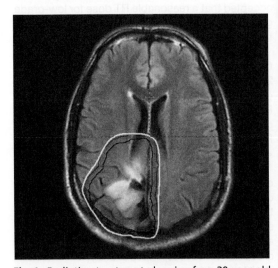

Fig. 1. Radiation treatment planning for a 29-year-old man with a right parietal lobe oligodendroglioma, World Health Organization grade II, who underwent active surveillance after surgery. He presented with radiographic evidence of disease progression 2 years from surgery and underwent radiotherapy of 5400 cGy in 200 cGy daily fractions with concurrent temozolomide. Note the T2 fluid-attenuated inversion recovery MRI sequence with hyperintensity. Clinical target volume (*blue*) and planning target volume (*red*) as well as the prescriptions are isodose (*yellow*).

alone in NCT 00313729) versus 10.4 years in the CRT arm (significantly superior to TMZ first).[8] The median overall survival with TMZ first in NCT 00313729 was 9.7 years compared with 7.8 years with RT alone in RTOG 9802, but significantly lower than the 13.3 years achieved with RT plus PCV in RTOG 9802. It is, therefore, our contention that the current standard of care is and should be RT plus PCV until it is bested.

Although RTOG 9802 showed the benefit of PCV chemotherapy, it remains unclear whether TMZ, which is easier to administer and commonly used for high-grade gliomas, is just as efficacious as PCV. There have been no randomized trials for low-grade glioma directly comparing TMZ with PCV. The best available data on TMZ in a clinical trial for WHO grade II gliomas comes from RTOG 0424, a multicenter phase II trial for patients with high-risk low-grade glioma as defined by Pignatti and colleagues,[3] which combined RT to 54 Gy with concurrent and adjuvant TMZ.[18] In a preliminary analysis, the 3-year overall survival rate was 73.1%, which was higher than historical controls and the study's hypothesized rate of 65%.

Additional long-term data will be required to assess long-term efficacy of TMZ and RT for low-grade glioma.

TECHNOLOGICAL ADVANCES OF RADIOTHERAPY: INTENSITY-MODULATED RADIOTHERAPY, PROTON THERAPY, AND CARBON THERAPY

Because patients with low-grade glioma may live for many years, it is important not only to improve survival outcomes, but also to minimize RT-related late effects. Advances in RT delivery systems allow for more conformal radiation treatment planning to maximize RT doses to target volumes while minimizing dose to surrounding normal structures. Intensity-modulated RT has been frequently used for the treatment of adult and pediatric brain tumors and in many studies reported to offer improved conformity than traditional 3-dimensional conformal radiotherapy techniques (**Figs. 1** and **2**).[19–29] Importantly, intensity-modulated RT has the ability to decrease the dose to surrounding critical structures, such as the

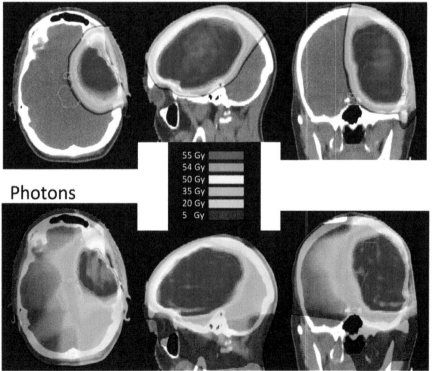

Protons

Photons

55 Gy	
54 Gy	
50 Gy	
35 Gy	
20 Gy	
5 Gy	

Fig. 2. Dosimetric plans of proton therapy versus photon therapy for a low-grade glioma of the left temporal lobe are shown. Equivalent tumor target dose coverage is achieved, but markedly less radiation is delivered to nontarget tissues with proton therapy. (*From* Shih HA, Sherman JC, Nachtigall LB, et al. Proton therapy for low-grade gliomas: results from a prospective trial. Cancer 2015;121(10):1713; with permission.)

Table 2
Ongoing phase III randomized trials for radiotherapy for low-grade gliomas

Trial	ClinicalTrials.gov Identifier	Treatment Arm
NRG-BN005[a]	NCT03180502	54 Gy (photons) with adjuvant temozolomide 54 Gy (protons) with adjuvant temozolomide
Adjuvant Temozolomide for Low Grade Glioma (China)	NCT01649830	54 Gy 54 Gy with adjuvant temozolomide
ECOG-E3F05	NCT00978458	50.4 Gy 50.4 Gy with adjuvant temozolomide

[a] Includes intermediate/anaplastic gliomas.

cochlea and hippocampus, and is associated with decreased ototoxicity and neurotoxicity rates.[27,30,31]

Although intensity-modulated RT has dosimetric advantages over 3-dimensional conformal radiotherapy, the advantages of proton therapy and carbon therapy are being investigated. One of the earliest experiences of proton therapy for low-grade glioma was a small series of 19 patients treated with protons in Germany demonstrating low toxicity rates, comparable with photon-based radiotherapy.[32] A pooled analysis of several proton centers found no grade III or higher side effects in patients with low-grade glioma, but did report frequent grade I and II acute toxicities, including alopecia (81%), fatigue (47%), and headaches (40%).[33] Sherman and colleagues[34] reported a small cohort of 20 patients with low-grade glioma treated with proton therapy who were evaluated prospectively with comprehensive neuropsychological testing. At a median follow-up of 5 years, the authors report that patients exhibited stable posttreatment cognitive functioning and that tumor location was associated with neurocognitive performance. Interestingly, patients with left hemispheric tumors were more impaired versus those with tumors in the right hemisphere. A separate analysis from Shih and colleagues[35] found that 20 patients with low-grade glioma who underwent proton therapy experienced a 3-year progression-free survival of 85%, which decreased to 40% at 5 years (**Fig. 2**). These results suggest that proton therapy may provide neurocognitive advantages over photons but may not confer overall or progression-free survival advantages. Ongoing trials randomizing patients with low-grade glioma to protons versus photons will help us to understand whether protons may provide improved neurocognitive preservation.

ONGOING RADIOTHERAPY TRIALS FOR LOW-GRADE GLIOMA

Based on the results of previously discussed studies, ongoing trials are now comparing photons versus protons and evaluating the role of adjuvant TMZ (**Table 2**). NRG-BN005 (NCT03180502) is a phase II randomized trial of proton versus photon therapy for IDH-mutant low- and intermediate-grade gliomas using 54 Gy. The primary endpoint is to assess whether proton therapy preserves cognitive outcomes over time as measured by the Clinical Trial Battery Composite score, which is calculated from the Hopkins Verbal Learning Test Revised Total and Delayed Recall, Controlled Oral Word association Test, and Trail Making Test Parts A and B. It should be noted that patients with WHO grade III IDH-mutant glioma may be enrolled in this trial. ECOG-E3F05 (NCT00978458) is a phase III trial randomizing low-grade glioma patents with uncontrolled symptoms, tumor progression, or age of 40 years or greater to 50.4 Gy of RT with concurrent and adjuvant TMZ versus 50.4 Gy RT alone. The primary endpoint is to determine whether the addition of TMZ improves progression-free survival and/or overall survival. A similar phase III trial in China (NCT01649830) is randomizing patients with low-grade glioma to 54 Gy RT with or without adjuvant TMZ.

SUMMARY

Recent studies have broadened our understanding of both the diagnosis and treatment of low-grade glioma. Molecular biomarkers play a vital role in the prognostication of low-grade glioma. Treatment options for low-grade glioma include surgery, observation (in highly selected subsets), radiotherapy, and/or chemotherapy. The preponderance of data suggest that, for those needing either RT or chemotherapy, the combination is the superior approach. Treatment decisions including RT must consider all prognostic factors including molecular biomarkers and weigh both the long-term benefits and risks of RT. Patients with high-risk low-grade gliomas should be considered for early adjuvant RT. Long-term results and additional studies are needed to address the role of adjuvant TMZ combined with RT and the benefits of advanced RT technologies, such as protons and carbon ion therapy.

REFERENCES

1. Youland RS, Schomas DA, Brown PD, et al. Changes in presentation, treatment, and outcomes of adult low-grade gliomas over the past fifty years. Neuro Oncol 2013;15(8):1102–10.
2. Louis DN, Perry A, Reifenberger G, et al. The 2016 World Health Organization Classification of Tumors of the Central Nervous System: a summary. Acta Neuropathol 2016;131(6):803–20.
3. Pignatti F, van den Bent M, Curran D, et al. Prognostic factors for survival in adult patients with cerebral low-grade glioma. J Clin Oncol 2002;20(8): 2076–84.
4. Cancer Genome Atlas Research Network, Brat DJ, Verhaak RG, et al. Comprehensive, integrative genomic analysis of diffuse lower-grade gliomas. N Engl J Med 2015;372(26):2481–98.
5. Eckel-Passow JE, Lachance DH, Molinaro AM, et al. Glioma groups based on 1p/19q, IDH, and TERT promoter mutations in tumors. N Engl J Med 2015; 372(26):2499–508.
6. Jenkins RB, Blair H, Ballman KV, et al. A t(1;19)(q10; p10) mediates the combined deletions of 1p and 19q and predicts a better prognosis of patients with oligodendroglioma. Cancer Res 2006;66(20): 9852–61.
7. Reuss DE, Kratz A, Sahm F, et al. Adult IDH wild type astrocytomas biologically and clinically resolve into other tumor entities. Acta Neuropathol 2015;130(3): 407–17.
8. Buckner JC, Shaw EG, Pugh SL, et al. Radiation plus procarbazine, CCNU, and vincristine in low-grade glioma. N Engl J Med 2016;374(14): 1344–55.
9. Sun H, Yin L, Li S, et al. Prognostic significance of IDH mutation in adult low-grade gliomas: a meta-analysis. J Neurooncol 2013;113(2):277–84.
10. Shaw E, Arusell R, Scheithauer B, et al. Prospective randomized trial of low- versus high-dose radiation therapy in adults with supratentorial low-grade glioma: initial report of a North Central Cancer Treatment Group/Radiation Therapy Oncology Group/ Eastern Cooperative Oncology Group study. J Clin Oncol 2002;20(9):2267–76.
11. Brown PD, Buckner JC, O'Fallon JR, et al. Effects of radiotherapy on cognitive function in patients with low-grade glioma measured by the Folstein mini-mental state examination. J Clin Oncol 2003; 21(13):2519–24.
12. Karim AB, Maat B, Hatlevoll R, et al. A randomized trial on dose-response in radiation therapy of low-grade cerebral glioma: European Organization for Research and Treatment of Cancer (EORTC) Study 22844. Int J Radiat Oncol Biol Phys 1996;36(3): 549–56.
13. van den Bent MJ, Afra D, de Witte O, et al. Long-term efficacy of early versus delayed radiotherapy for low-grade astrocytoma and oligodendroglioma in adults: the EORTC 22845 randomised trial. Lancet 2005;366(9490):985–90.
14. Shaw EG, Berkey B, Coons SW, et al. Recurrence following neurosurgeon-determined gross-total resection of adult supratentorial low-grade glioma: results of a prospective clinical trial. J Neurosurg 2008;109(5):835–41.
15. Baumert BG, Hegi ME, van den Bent MJ, et al. Temozolomide chemotherapy versus radiotherapy in high-risk low-grade glioma (EORTC 22033-26033): a randomised, open-label, phase 3 intergroup study. Lancet Oncol 2016;17(11):1521–32.
16. Reijneveld JC, Taphoorn MJ, Coens C, et al. Health-related quality of life in patients with high-risk low-grade glioma (EORTC 22033-26033): a randomised, open-label, phase 3 intergroup study. Lancet Oncol 2016;17(11):1533–42.
17. Wahl M, Phillips JJ, Molinaro AM, et al. Chemotherapy for adult low-grade gliomas: clinical outcomes by molecular subtype in a phase II study of adjuvant temozolomide. Neuro Oncol 2017;19(2): 242–51.
18. Fisher BJ, Hu C, Macdonald DR, et al. Phase 2 study of temozolomide-based chemoradiation therapy for high-risk low-grade gliomas: preliminary results of Radiation Therapy Oncology Group 0424. Int J Radiat Oncol Biol Phys 2015; 91(3):497–504.
19. Aherne NJ, Benjamin LC, Horsley PJ, et al. Improved outcomes with intensity modulated radiation therapy combined with temozolomide for newly diagnosed glioblastoma multiforme. Neurol Res Int 2014;2014:945620.
20. Amelio D, Lorentini S, Schwarz M, et al. Intensity-modulated radiation therapy in newly diagnosed glioblastoma: a systematic review on clinical and technical issues. Radiother Oncol 2010;97(3): 361–9.
21. Burnet NG, Jena R, Burton KE, et al. Clinical and practical considerations for the use of intensity-modulated radiotherapy and image guidance in neuro-oncology. Clin Oncol (R Coll Radiol) 2014; 26(7):395–406.

22. Chan MF, Schupak K, Burman C, et al. Comparison of intensity-modulated radiotherapy with three-dimensional conformal radiation therapy planning for glioblastoma multiforme. Med Dosim 2003; 28(4):261–5.

23. Hermanto U, Frija EK, Lii MJ, et al. Intensity-modulated radiotherapy (IMRT) and conventional three-dimensional conformal radiotherapy for high-grade gliomas: does IMRT increase the integral dose to normal brain? Int J Radiat Oncol Biol Phys 2007; 67(4):1135–44.

24. Navarria P, Pessina F, Cozzi L, et al. Can advanced new radiation therapy technologies improve outcome of high grade glioma (HGG) patients? analysis of 3D-conformal radiotherapy (3DCRT) versus volumetric-modulated arc therapy (VMAT) in patients treated with surgery, concomitant and adjuvant chemo-radiotherapy. BMC Cancer 2016;16:362.

25. Paulino AC, Lobo M, Teh BS, et al. Ototoxicity after intensity-modulated radiation therapy and cisplatin-based chemotherapy in children with medulloblastoma. Int J Radiat Oncol Biol Phys 2010;78(5): 1445–50.

26. Paulino AC, Mazloom A, Terashima K, et al. Intensity-modulated radiotherapy (IMRT) in pediatric low-grade glioma. Cancer 2013;119(14):2654–9.

27. Polkinghorn WR, Dunkel IJ, Souweidane MM, et al. Disease control and ototoxicity using intensity-modulated radiation therapy tumor-bed boost for medulloblastoma. Int J Radiat Oncol Biol Phys 2011;81(3):e15–20.

28. Schroeder TM, Chintagumpala M, Okcu MF, et al. Intensity-modulated radiation therapy in childhood ependymoma. Int J Radiat Oncol Biol Phys 2008; 71(4):987–93.

29. Yang Z, Zhang Z, Wang X, et al. Intensity-modulated radiotherapy for gliomas: dosimetric effects of changes in gross tumor volume on organs at risk and healthy brain tissue. Onco Targets Ther 2016; 9:3545–54.

30. Gondi V, Pugh SL, Tome WA, et al. Preservation of memory with conformal avoidance of the hippocampal neural stem-cell compartment during whole-brain radiotherapy for brain metastases (RTOG 0933): a phase II multi-institutional trial. J Clin Oncol 2014;32(34):3810–6.

31. Vieira WA, Weltman E, Chen MJ, et al. Ototoxicity evaluation in medulloblastoma patients treated with involved field boost using intensity-modulated radiation therapy (IMRT): a retrospective review. Radiat Oncol 2014;9:158.

32. Hauswald H, Rieken S, Ecker S, et al. First experiences in treatment of low-grade glioma grade I and II with proton therapy. Radiat Oncol 2012;7:189.

33. Wilkinson B, Morgan H, Gondi V, et al. Low levels of acute toxicity associated with proton therapy for low-grade glioma: a proton collaborative group study. Int J Radiat Oncol Biol Phys 2016;96(2S):E135.

34. Sherman JC, Colvin MK, Mancuso SM, et al. Neurocognitive effects of proton radiation therapy in adults with low-grade glioma. J Neurooncol 2016;126(1): 157–64.

35. Shih HA, Sherman JC, Nachtigall LB, et al. Proton therapy for low-grade gliomas: results from a prospective trial. Cancer 2015;121(10):1712–9.

Higher-Order Surgical Questions for Diffuse Low-Grade Gliomas
Supramaximal Resection, Neuroplasticity, and Screening

Hugues Duffau, MD, PhD[a,b,*]

KEYWORDS

- Diffuse low-grade glioma • Awake mapping • Quality of life • Brain remapping • Screening
- Neuroplasticity • Connectomics

KEY POINTS

- Early and maximal safe surgical resection of diffuse low-grade glioma (DLGG) by means of awake mapping allows a significant improvement of survival and quality of life.
- Supramarginal removal of DLGG seems to minimize the risk of malignant transformation of DLGG.
- Neuroplasticity is valuable to resect DLGG in critical brain structures, possibly in several surgeries, in order to use functional remapping over time.
- It is time to move toward a screening in the general population, with the aim to develop a prophylactic surgical neuro-oncology.

INTRODUCTION

Supratentorial diffuse low-grade glioma (DLGG) is a primary brain tumor that generally occurs in young adults who enjoyed an active life, initially with no or only mild functional disorders.[1] This neoplasm is most often diagnosed because of seizures, even though incidental discovery is becoming increasingly frequent. DLGG progresses continuously, invades the connectome by migrating along the white matter fibers, and inescapably becomes a high-grade glioma if left untreated. Such a malignant transformation leads to neurocognitive and/or neurologic deteriorations, and ultimately to the death.[2] In series in which early radical surgery was not performed, the overall survival (OS) was approximately 6 to 7 years.[3,4] Remarkably, in the modern literature, a large amount of data demonstrated that surgical removal performed at diagnosis impacted significantly the natural course of DLGG, in particular when the resection objectively calculated on postoperative T2/fluid-attenuated inversion recovery (FLAIR)-weighted MRI was total or at least subtotal (namely, <10–15 mL of residue).[5–7] In fact, in experiences based on precocious and maximal surgery, OS is approximately 13 to 15 years, thereby doubling the survival in comparison with a wait-and-see attitude.[8–10]

Disclosure Statement: The author has nothing to declare.
[a] Department of Neurosurgery, Gui de Chauliac Hospital, CHU Montpellier, Montpellier University Medical Center, 80, Avenue Augustin Fliche, Montpellier 34295, France; [b] Team "Plasticity of Central Nervous System, Human Stem Cells and Glial Tumors", Institute for Neuroscience of Montpellier, INSERM U1051, Saint Eloi Hospital, Montpellier University Medical Center, Montpellier, France
* Department of Neurosurgery, Gui de Chauliac Hospital, CHU Montpellier, 80, Avenue Augustin Fliche, Montpellier 34295, France.
E-mail address: h-duffau@chu-montpellier.fr

Neurosurg Clin N Am 30 (2019) 119–128
https://doi.org/10.1016/j.nec.2018.08.009
1042-3680/19/© 2018 Elsevier Inc. All rights reserved.

Thus, early radical excision is nowadays the first treatment in patients with DLGG, on condition that the quality of life (QoL) is preserved.[1,11,12]

In this spirit, due to a major anatomo-functional variability of brain organization across individuals, intraoperative mapping has been increasingly used for DLGG surgery, especially in awake patients. The principle is based on the use of direct electrostimulation (DES) to map the cortical-subcortical structures, combined with online neurocognitive monitoring throughout the resection, with the aim of detecting the critical neural circuits. This allows the identification and preservation of both the cortex and the white matter tracts that are essential for brain processes at the individual level, on the basis of real-time structural-functional correlations performed with a great accuracy and reproducibility.[13] As shown by a meta-analysis based on more than 8000 gliomas, DES mapping resulted in significantly reducing the rate of severe persistent deficits, even in so-called "eloquent regions," while increasing the extent of resection (EOR).[14] In large series of awake surgery for gliomas, fewer than 2% of permanent deteriorations have been generated.[15–17] In other words, with awake mapping, it is now possible to optimize the onco-functional balance in patients with DLGG, by enabling them to live longer and better.[12]

However, despite these considerable advances, several higher-order surgical questions remain unsolved. First, most of DLGGs will recur, even following a complete resection objectively demonstrated on the postoperative MRI. Additionally, although neuroplasticity makes possible surgery for DLGG located in areas classically considered as unresectable, it is nonetheless not rare to be obliged to leave a residue when the tumor involves neural networks still crucial for brain functioning. This is particularly true when the glioma is already voluminous or very diffuse, a common occurrence in patients with preoperative neurologic impairment. Here, the goal is to propose new concepts to address these issues in DLGG, as follows: (1) when feasible, to evolve into the philosophy of supramarginal resection to prevent malignant transformation; (2) to use the neuroplastic potential to offer resection in "eloquent sites," knowing that, when a total removal was not possible during the first surgery, mechanisms of brain remapping over years can permit a reoperation with an improvement of the EOR; and (3) to propose a screening in the general population, with the aim of discovering smaller gliomas, and thus of increasing the chance of (supra)maximal resection, while preserving the QoL, even in asymptomatic patients.

SUPRAMAXIMAL RESECTION IN DIFFUSE LOW-GRADE GLIOMA: IS IT EFFECTIVE AND SAFE?

Supramaximal Resection in Diffuse Low-Grade Glioma is Effective

Biopsy samples revealed that conventional MRI underestimated the actual spatial extent of DLGG, because tumor cells were found beyond the area of signal abnormalities, up to 2 cm, even for gliomas well defined on MRI.[18] Therefore, it has been suggested that an extended surgical excision aimed at removing a security margin beyond these MRI-defined abnormalities, that is, a "supramaximal resection" (**Fig. 1**), might improve the oncological outcome.[19] In this way, a seminal experience showed that such a supratotal resection achieved in 15 patients bearing a DLGG within "noneloquent" cerebral regions prevented malignant transformation with a mean follow-up of 35.7 months (range 6–135).[20] This cohort was compared with a control group of 29 patients who benefited "only" from a total removal of a DLGG: although malignant transformation was observed in 7 cases in the control group, no degeneration occurred in patients who underwent supramarginal resection ($P = .037$). Moreover, adjuvant oncological therapy was administrated in 10 cases in the control group compared with only 1 case following supramaximal resection ($P = .043$).[20]

More recently, a study analyzed the long-term outcome (with a follow-up of 132 months, range, 97–198 months) after a supracomplete DLGG removal.[21] The resection was pursued until eloquent cortical and subcortical structures identified by intraoperative DES mapping were encountered. No chemotherapy or radiotherapy was given after resection. There was no recurrence in half of cases. Fifteen percent of patients experienced glioma relapse, with an average time of 70.3 months (range, 32–105 months): nonetheless, there was no malignant transformation. Therefore, this series demonstrated for the first time the prolonged impact of supramaximal surgery on DLGG, because removal of a safety margin around the tumor visible on MRI seems to minimize the risk of malignization.[21]

Of note, the 50% rate of recurrence is likely due to the impossibility to take enough margin all around the tumor for functional issues. Interestingly, in some patients, the relapse occurred after only 32 months, whereas in others, there was no recurrence with 198 months of follow-up after the sole surgery (no adjuvant treatment).[21] This might be because certain DLGGs are more "proliferative"

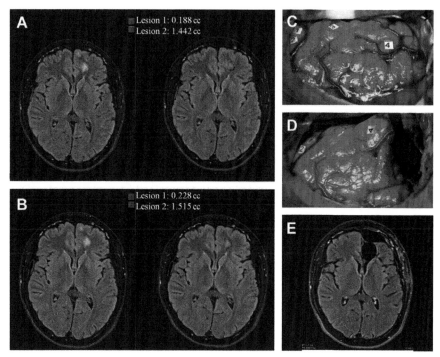

Fig. 1. (*A*) Axial FLAIR-weighted MRI showing 2 lesions compatible with a multicentric left frontal DLGG in a 27-year-old right-handed man, without any symptoms, who intentionally performed brain neuroimaging because his father died from a glioblastoma. The neurologic and neurocognitive examination was normal. (*B*) Axial FLAIR-weighted MRI performed 6 months after the first imaging, demonstrating an objective growth of both lesions thanks to an objective volumetric assessment, supporting the diagnosis of iDLGG. Therefore, surgery was proposed to the patient. (*C*) Intraoperative view before resection in awake patient. The anterior part of the right hemisphere is on the left and its posterior part is on the right. Number tags show zones of positive DES mapping. (*D*) Intraoperative view after functional-based resection in awake patient. The surgical removal was pursued until DES mapping detected eloquent neural structures, both at cortical and subcortical levels. (*E*) Postoperative FLAIR-weighted MRI, demonstrating a supracomplete resection. The patient resumed a normal familial, social, and professional life within 3 months after surgery, with an improvement of scores in some neurocognitive domains in comparison with the presurgical status, as evidenced by an objective neuropsychological assessment performed after a postoperative functional rehabilitation.

(with more sharp borders on MRI), whereas other DLGGs are more "invasive" (with more indistinct borders on MRI): these patterns seem at least in part be related to the molecular profile, because bulky DLGGs are more frequently isocitrate dehydrogenase (IDH)-mutant, whereas tumors with indistinct limits are more often IDH wild-type and 1p19q non-codeleted.[22] Supramaximal resection has likely a better chance of controlling for a long time the former than the latter pattern. Advances in metabolic imaging, closer to the actual glioma infiltration, as validated by coregistration of histologic and radiological characteristics,[23] could enable a better selection of indications for supracomplete resection. Another helpful method might be the biomathematical models of proliferation and diffusion, based on at least 2 sets of MRI scans acquired 3 to 6 months apart, before any treatment.[24]

Supramaximal Resection in Diffuse Low-Grade Glioma is Safe

Supramarginal resection of DLGG does not burden the QoL. Indeed, in the 2 first series reported, no permanent neurologic worsening has been observed, and all patients resumed a normal familial, social, and professional life.[20,21] This is due to the use of awake mapping by means of DES, even for tumors involving area traditionally regarded as "noneloquent." In fact, besides the classic motor and language mapping, it is also crucial to spare the neural networks underpinning higher-order cognitive and behavioral functions in supratotal removal, because, in essence, the resection is achieved up to functional boundaries.[13] To this end, additional tasks have been implemented for the intraoperative monitoring, including when surgery is performed in the right "nondominant" hemisphere,[25,26] to preserve an optimal QoL redefined at the individual level, according to the job, hobbies, and lifestyle of each patient. In practice, it is nowadays possible to map a panel of brain functions, such as reading, calculation, complex movement (eg, bimanual co-ordination), visuo-spatial cognition, verbal and nonverbal semantics, judgment, memory, attentional processing, and even theory of mind.[27] The selection of appropriate tasks should be made not only based on the brain topography of the tumor but also on the basis of the patient's needs. Thanks to this paradigm shift from image-guided resection to functional-based resection of diffuse gliomas, with the integration during surgery of more sensitive tests allowing the mapping of subtle functions, the outcome after maximal DLGG removal has been improved. Indeed, beyond the fact that the rate of permanent neurologic impairments has significantly decreased (nil in a recent prospective cohort of 374 awake craniotomies[17]), objective postoperative neuropsychological assessments have demonstrated that higher-order brain functions, such as semantic processing, attention, working memory, mentalizing, or metacognition, were preserved and even improved after large DLGG excision.[28–31]

To sum up, the aim of supramarginal resection is to prevent malignant transformation for a prolonged period (at least 1 to 2 decades) by reducing the number of peripheral tumoral cells as well as to postpone adjuvant therapy, while preserving a normal QoL. However, one cannot (yet) claim to cure patients with DLGG, except possibly in selected cases with a more "proliferative" pattern and with an early diagnosis that permitted removing at least 2 cm of safety margin all around the neoplasm. This is the reason why consideration may be given to screening in the general population, because the rate of supraradical removal is higher in incidental DLGG (see later in this article).[32]

WHEN TO USE PLASTICITY TO MAXIMIZE EXTENT OF RESECTION IN DIFFUSE LOW-GRADE GLIOMA?
The Role of Brain Reallocation in Surgery for Diffuse Low-Grade Glioma Within Eloquent Areas

Recent advances in cognitive neurosciences have resulted in a revisitation of models underlying cerebral processing, that is, a switch from the rigid localist view to a networking organization of the human brain. In this dynamic framework, neural functions are subserved by the interaction and integration of large-scale parallel subcircuits able to compensate themselves, at least to a certain extent. Such a connectomal account opens the door to mechanisms of neuroplasticity, which are frequent in cases of slow-growing lesions such as DLGG.[33] This explains why patients with DLGG usually lead a normal life at diagnosis, even though slight cognitive disturbances may be observed when an accurate neuropsychological evaluation is achieved before any therapy: in other words, the neuroplastic potential is considerable but it has nonetheless limitations. In our recent atlas of brain plasticity, built on the basis of data gained from intraoperative DES mapping, the main limits of neural remodeling were represented by the white matter tracts (especially the superior longitudinal fascicle and arcuate fascicle complex mediating the dorsal stream, as well as the inferior fronto-occipital fascicle underpinning the ventral semantic stream), in addition to the input (as the visual system) and the output (as the primary motor system).[34,35] As a consequence, although the interindividual anatomo-functional variability is huge at the cortical level, due to the high plastic potential of the cortex, the variability is reduced at the subcortical level, due to the low plastic potential of the axonal fibers.[36]

In surgical practice, the implication of functional reshaping is very important, because this dynamic potential makes possible resection in "eloquent" regions such as the Broca area, Wernicke area, Rolandic area, or the insula without inducing any persistent neurologic deterioration.[37] Such results should provide an incentive to propose in a more systematic manner surgical removal for DLGG involving structures deemed "unresectable" in a fixed and localizationist model of brain processes, in particular based on imaging studies.[38] In fact, despite a transitory worsening in the immediate postoperative period, patients will recover thanks to the identification and preservation of critical neural pathways by means of DES mapping (see earlier in this article),[13] combined with postoperative functional rehabilitation.[39] Recent studies using presurgical and postsurgical functional neuroimaging have shown a reorganization of the cerebral networks, with recruitment of perilesional and remote brain epicenters localized in both hemispheres and interconnected by white matter fibers.[40,41] For example, resting-state functional MRI has been performed before, during, and after a supplementary motor area (SMA) syndrome transiently generated by surgery for DLGG involving the frontomesial structures.[42] The results evidenced a large-scale reshaping of the sensorimotor network. Interhemispheric connectivity was decreased in the postoperative period, when the patient experienced the transient SMA syndrome, and increased again during the recovery process. Indeed, connectivity between the ipsilesional motor area and the contralateral SMA rose to higher values than in the preoperative period. In addition, intrahemispheric connectivity was decreased during the immediate postoperative period and had returned to preoperative values at 3 months following DLGG resection.[42] Longitudinal changes in cerebellar and thalamic spontaneous activity have also been observed before and after surgery by means of resting-state functional MRI.[41] In the same way, in DLGG within the right hemisphere, an impressive reallocation of networks mediating visuospatial attention, has been found using preoperative and postoperative diffusion tensor imaging tractography, with a crucial role of the contralateral left hemisphere and of the long-range white matter pathways in the right hemisphere.[30] This supports the preservation of the subcortical connectivity at the end of surgical resection, owing to the use of axonal DES.[27]

The Value of Functional Remapping for a Multistage Surgical Strategy in Diffuse Low-Grade Glioma

As mentioned, because of the invasive feature of DLGG, tumor recurrence is possible following total or even supratotal resection, knowing that a constant progression of the residual glioma is, in essence, inevitable after incomplete removal. In this context, several reports have demonstrated the oncological impact of reoperation(s) in DLGG. Beyond the fact that a greater initial EOR was prognostic for time to reintervention,[43] a series with 130 DLGGs showed that extended resection for nonmalignant relapse (a complete removal could be performed in 53.1% of recurrent tumors) increased the OS significantly.[44] In the experience of the French Glioma Consortium, subsequent surgical removal was an independent prognostic factor significantly correlated with a longer OS.[8] Furthermore, in a consecutive series of DLGG with reoperation for tumor recurrence in eloquent areas, a total or subtotal resection was achieved in 73.7% of cases during the reintervention, despite an involvement of critical structures. This means that a "multistep surgical approach," with a first maximal function-based resection, followed by a period of several years, and then a reintervention with an increase of EOR while preserving QoL, can be conceived because of phenomena of functional reshaping induced by the glioma (re)growth, by the first resection itself, and by postoperative rehabilitation (**Fig. 2**).[45]

In this state of mind, in a study with 18 patients who benefited from repeat awake craniotomy for glioma with a mean interval between surgical procedures of 4.1 years, intraoperative mapping revealed functional plasticity. Indeed, during intraoperative DES, one-third of patients exhibited loss of function at 1 or more motor or language areas between surgeries, with no neurologic deterioration, suggesting that brain function was preserved through neural remodeling or activation of latent functional networks.[46] Consequently, at reoperation, an updated remapping is highly mandatory. More recently, a series of 42 patients with DLGG who underwent iterative awake surgeries with DES mapping (mean interval between surgical procedures of 4.5 years), showed that the patterns of functional reshaping may differ between patients, resulting in an individual-specific reorganized brain.[47] In fact, cortical mappings exhibited a high level of plasticity (displacement of ≥ 2 sites) in 23 patients, whereas there was a low level of plasticity in the 19 other cases. Remarkably, more efficient plasticity mechanisms are facilitated by cortical and bulky tumors, and they are associated with an increase of EOR at reoperation and with earlier functional recovery. This means that tumoral invasion of the white matter tracts represents the main limitation of neuroplastic potential: this connectomal constraint limits EOR during the second surgery. Therefore, because axonal plasticity is low, if glioma progression after the first surgery exhibits a very diffuse pattern with considerable migration along the subcortical fibers, adjuvant oncological therapy can be considered rather than to propose subsequent surgery, which will not be able to improve EOR. In contrast, in cases of recurrent DLGG mainly involving the cortex and with more sharp borders on MRI, a second (or even a third) awake surgery should be envisioned more systematically, before the onset of malignant transformation, with the goal to improve both OS and QoL.[47] In other words, it is currently possible to tailor a multistage therapeutic strategy at the individual level according to the pattern of tumor progression and to the reactional adaptation of the central nervous system.

SCREENING: WHAT TO DO WITH INCIDENTAL DIFFUSE LOW-GRADE GLIOMA?
Incidental Diffuse Low-Grade Glioma Exhibits a Similar Natural History to Symptomatic Diffuse Low-Grade Glioma

Thanks to a facilitated access to neuroimaging worldwide, incidental DLGG (iDLGG) can be increasingly discovered on an MRI performed for

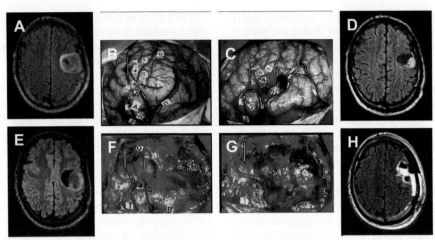

Fig. 2. (*A*) Preoperative axial FLAIR-weighted MRI revealing a left premotor DLGG in a 24-year-old right-handed man who experienced seizures. The neurologic and neurocognitive examination was normal. (*B*) Intraoperative view before resection in awake patient. The anterior part of the left hemisphere is on the right and its posterior part is on the left. Tumor borders were marked with letter tags. Number tags show zones of positive DES mapping. 1, 2, 3: primary motor cortex of the right upper limb, generating involuntary movement of the right arm/hand during DES; 4, 5, 6: ventral premotor cortex, inducing anarthria during DES. Long arrow: central sulcus; short arrow: precentral sulcus. (*C*) Intraoperative view after functional-based resection in awake patient. The surgical removal was pursued until DES mapping detected eloquent neural structures, both at cortical and subcortical levels. Short arrow: precentral sulcus. (*D*) Postoperative FLAIR-weighted MRI, demonstrating an incomplete resection, with a residue voluntarily left in the premotor cortex to avoid permanent deficit. The patient resumed a normal familial, social, and professional life within 3 months after surgery. The diagnosis of Wordl Health Organization (WHO) grade II glioma was histologically confirmed. No adjuvant treatment was given. (*E*) Axial FLAIR-weighted MRI showing a significant growth (18 mL) of the residual tumor 10 years after the first surgery in a patient with a neurologic and neurocognitive examination still normal. However, due to the recent onset of seizures (although the patient had no epilepsy for 9 years), reoperation was proposed. (*F*) Intraoperative view before resection in awake patient. The anterior part of the left hemisphere is on the right and its posterior part is on the left. Tumor borders were marked with letter tags. Number tags show zones of positive direct electrostimulation mapping, with identification of the primary motor cortex of the upper limb (1, 2, 3, 4), as during the first surgery, but with no functional responses during DES of the ventral premotor cortex, revealing a remapping in comparison with the previous DES mapping achieved 10 years ago. Long arrow: central sulcus; short arrow: precentral sulcus. (*G*) Intraoperative view after functional-based resection in awake patient. The surgical removal was pursued until DES mapping detected eloquent neural structures, both at cortical and subcortical levels (50: anterior part of the superior longitudinal fasciculus, eliciting phonological disorders during DES; 49: anterior part of the inferior fronto-occipital fasciculus, generating semantic disorders during DES). Interestingly, the ventral premotor region was removed, allowing an optimization of the EOR compared with the first surgical excision, thanks to functional reshaping. Arrow: central sulcus. (*H*) Postoperative FLAIR-weighted MRI, demonstrating a complete resection. The patient resumed a normal familial, social, and professional life within 3 months after surgery, with no more epilepsy. The tumor was still a WHO grade II glioma according to the neuropathological examination. No adjuvant oncological treatment was administered.

other reasons, mainly head injury, unrelated headaches or dizziness, follow-up of another cerebral lesion, or participation in a research protocol. Although these patients could be thought of as asymptomatic in the context of incidental diagnosis, it has recently been demonstrated in a series focusing on patients with iDLGG that they actually did suffer from neuropsychological disorders.[48] Indeed, by asking them to describe the difficulties encountered in the previous year and by achieving an objective neurocognitive assessment before treatment, two-thirds of patients with iDLGG reported subjective complaints, mostly tiredness (40%) and attention disturbances (33%), with impairment of neurocognitive functions in 60% of cases: 53% with altered executive functions, 20% with working memory deficits, and 6% with attention disorders.[48] This means that a neuropsychological evaluation must be performed in a more systematic way in iDLGG due to the high prevalence of insidious cognitive deficits. Furthermore, these findings raise into question the classic wait-and-watch attitude in iDLGG, mainly based on the erroneous dogma that these patients have no functional deteriorations.

From a radiological point of view, by measuring the growth rate computed from the volumetric assessment of iDLGG on repeat MRIs 3 to 6 months apart, a constant linear progression of the mean diameter approximately 3.5 to 4.0 mm per year has been calculated, that is, similar to the velocity diametric expansion calculated in symptomatic DLGG.[49] Such an objective demonstration of progression of the signal abnormality should be evidenced before to propose any treatment, especially surgical excision. Indeed, although the diagnosis can be easy when the morphologic and metabolic aspect on MRI is typical, it could be more difficult in other conditions, particularly for small lesions. In an experience with 72 patients with suspected iDLGG, due to a strict radiological stability for more than 5 years in 15 cases, the diagnosis of glioma was rejected.[50] In practice, an initial radiological follow-up is always needed, in agreement with 2 series that investigated the natural history of iDLGG, and that reported a median time between the first MRI and the oncological treatment of 10.4 and 21.0 months, respectively.[49,51]

In this setting, it is crucial to understand the functional and oncological consequences of the "silent" progression of iDLGG. First, from a functional point of view, glioma migration along the white matter tracts, which represents the limitation of neuroplastic potential as previously detailed,[33–35] will generate neurocognitive deficits; for example, verbal semantic disorders related to the invasion of the inferior fronto-occipital fasciculus[52] or mentalizing deterioration correlated to the infiltration of the arcuate fasciculus.[53] The next step will be the onset of seizures, meaning that the threshold of neural compensation has been reached.[54] The French Glioma Consortium showed that patients with iDLGG will become symptomatic following a median delay of 48 months.[49] Of note, if surgery is performed at that time, namely, when plasticity is already overpassed, resection will be most likely subtotal, with less chance to be total or supratotal. From an oncological point of view, the cumulative risk of malignization is increasing during the silent growth and migration. Such a progression to a higher grade, including acute malignization of iDLGG toward a glioblastoma, may occur despite an active surveillance, without the occurrence of any symptoms that could have acted as a warning to the physician.[55] In the same vein, microfoci of anaplasia have been a posteriori detected in 27% of patients who underwent surgery for an iDLGG.[56]

Surgery for Incidental Diffuse Low-Grade Glioma Is Safe While Improving the Extent of Resection

Because the lack of symptoms in patients with iDLGG does not protect from malignant transformation, and because (supra)marginal resection significantly increases OS by delaying such a degeneration in DLGG (see previously), "preventive" surgery has recently been proposed in iDLGG. Indeed, in symptomatic patients, supracomplete resections are rarely possible because the subcortical connectivity is already invaded in most patients. As mentioned, the ultimate aim in each case is to optimize the onco-functional balance, thus avoiding surgical damage to the white matter pathways to preserve the patient's functional status.[12,27] Remarkably, in 1 surgical series of iDLGG, because the tumor volumes were smaller than in symptomatic DLGGs, the rate of supratotal removals were much higher than for symptomatic patients.[56,57] In addition, QoL has been preserved, because none of the patients with iDLGG who underwent awake surgery by means of DES mapping experienced persistent neurologic impairments, and all patients resumed their work.[56] Furthermore, no long-lasting seizures have been observed in a recent surgical series of 21 patients for an iDLGG.[57] Consequently, given that a high rate of untreated patients with iDLGG already suffers from slight neurocognitive disturbances[48] and will experience epilepsy a few mo/y after diagnosis,[49] early surgical resection might contribute to delay such negative functional consequences by limiting the risk of diffusion of tumoral cells in neural networks that have not yet reached their limits of dynamic reorganization.[58] To sum up, these recent data support that prophylactic surgery in iDLGG with proven radiological growth may improve both OS and QoL.

Toward a Screening in the General Population

Due to the preliminary successes of the prophylactic surgery in patients with iDLGG, the idea of a screening in the general population has recently emerged.[59] First, it has been shown that the risk of overtreatment in case of incidental discovery of DLGG was low. Indeed, a recent investigation based on available epidemiologic data demonstrated that after an initial period of 4 years, the risk of dying from the silent iDLGG outweighed the risk of dying from another cause.[32] Second, a pilot survey revealed that 67% of healthy subjects were in favor of undergoing such a screening MRI.[60] Interestingly, this rate is in agreement with the proportion of people who effectively completed an MRI in the setting of a screening in a recent cohort with 2176 participants.[61] The prevalence of iDLGG in the general adult population has been estimated as approximately 4 per 10,000 in a meta-analysis of incidental findings on cerebral MRI.[62] It is worth noting this rate is much smaller than the proportion of other abnormal findings (approximately 3%), and that a categorization of incidental findings has recently been suggested.[61] Thus, if properly anticipated, the diagnosis of nonglioma abnormalities during screening is not an issue, on the condition that the patient is referred to an expert neurologist or neurosurgeon to discuss the different options regarding the discovered lesion.[63] Concerning the optimal timing of this screening, because recent series demonstrated using biomathematical modeling that the distribution of DLGG patient ages at the time of radiological onset had a Gaussian shape centered on 30 years of age, with a « width » of 10 years,[64] it has been proposed to screen at 20, 30, and 40 years of age.[65] Finally, from an economic point of view, a rough analysis has shown that the balance would be reached if one can gain 3 years of active life by screening and preventive treatment.[32] In clinical practice, there is a need to develop computational algorithms to detect automatically abnormal MRIs, knowing that sensitivity should prime over specificity, such that no abnormal MRIs would be missed.

Nonetheless, surgery for iDLGG should not only avoid any motor or language deteriorations, but also any deficits of cognitive, emotional, or social abilities, in young patients who are fully functional and socio-professionally active. In other words, in the context of intentional discovery, the bar must be set much higher in terms of functional results than in symptomatic patients (see **Fig. 1**). To this end, only ultraspecialized centers, integrating experts in neurosurgery, neuropsychology, neuroradiology, neuropathology, and neuro-oncology will likely obtain such results with a high level of reliability.[24]

SUMMARY

Surgical neuro-oncologists have to switch from the traditional approach of removing a DLGG tumor mass, to a multimodal and multistep surgical approach for a chronic tumoral disease, based on the understanding of the interactions between glioma progression and reactional cerebral remapping. The aim is to tailor a personalized management program according to the structural and functional organization of the connectome for a given patient at that time, and also to anticipate the next therapeutic stage by predicting how the central nervous system will reshape over mo/y. Therefore, brain surgeons must be first neuroscientists, to achieve earlier and more (supra) radical surgical resections of (incidentally/intentionally discovered) DLGG, owing to the mapping of neural networks and to the investigation of neuroplastic potential at the individual level. The ambitious goal of such prophylactic and functional surgical neuro-oncology is to optimize both OS and QoL in these usually young and active patients.

REFERENCES

1. Duffau H. Diffuse low-grade gliomas in adults: natural history, interaction with the brain, and new individualized therapeutic strategies. Duffau H, editor. 2nd edition. London: Springer; 2017.
2. Duffau H, Taillandier L. New concepts in the management of diffuse low-grade glioma: proposal of a multistage and individualized therapeutic approach. Neuro Oncol 2015;17:332–42.
3. Pignatti F, van den Bent M, Curran D, et al. Prognostic factors for survival in adult patients with cerebral low-grade glioma. J Clin Oncol 2002;20: 2076–84.
4. van den Bent MJ, Afra D, de Witte O, et al. Long-term efficacy of early versus delayed radiotherapy for low-grade astrocytoma and oligodendroglioma in adults: the EORTC 22845 randomised trial. Lancet 2005;366:985–90.
5. Smith JS, Chang EF, Lamborn KR, et al. Role of extent of resection in the long-term outcome of low-grade hemispheric gliomas. J Clin Oncol 2008; 26:1338–45.
6. Ius T, Isola M, Budai R, et al. Low-grade glioma surgery in eloquent areas: volumetric analysis of extent of resection and its impact on overall survival. A single-institution experience in 190 patients. J Neurosurg 2012;117:1039–52.
7. Roelz R, Strohmaier D, Jabbarli R, et al. Residual tumor volume as best outcome predictor in low grade glioma—a nine-years near-randomized survey of surgery vs. biopsy. Sci Rep 2016;6:32286.
8. Capelle L, Fontaine D, Mandonnet E, et al. Spontaneous and therapeutic prognostic factors in adult hemispheric WHO grade II gliomas: a series of 1097 cases. J Neurosurg 2013;118: 1157–68.
9. Jakola AS, Skjulsvik AJ, Myrmel KS, et al. Surgical resection versus watchful waiting in low-grade gliomas. Ann Oncol 2017;28:1942–8.
10. Pallud J, Audureau E, Blonski M, et al. Epileptic seizures in diffuse low-grade gliomas in adults. Brain 2014;137:449–62.
11. Soffietti R, Baumert B, Bello L, et al. Guidelines on management of low-grade gliomas: report of an

EFNS–EANO task force. Eur J Neurol 2010;17: 1124–33.

12. Mandonnet E, Duffau H. An attempt to conceptualize the individual onco-functional balance: why a standardized treatment is an illusion for diffuse low-grade glioma patients. Crit Rev Oncol Hematol 2018;122:83–91.

13. Duffau H. Resecting diffuse low-grade gliomas to the boundaries of brain functions: a new concept in surgical neuro-oncology. J Neurosurg Sci 2015; 59:361–71.

14. de Witt Hamer PC, Gil Robles S, Zwinderman A, et al. Impact of intraoperative stimulation brain mapping on glioma surgery outcome: a meta-analysis. J Clin Oncol 2012;30:2559–65.

15. Duffau H, Gatignol P, Mandonnet E, et al. Intraoperative subcortical stimulation mapping of language pathways in a consecutive series of 115 patients with Grade II glioma in the left dominant hemisphere. J Neurosurg 2008;109:461–71.

16. Sanai N, Mirzadeh Z, Berger MS. Functional outcome after language mapping for glioma resection. N Engl J Med 2008;358:18–27.

17. Boetto J, Bertram L, Moulinié G, et al. Low rate of intraoperative seizures during awake craniotomy in a prospective cohort with 374 supratentorial brain lesions: electrocorticography is not mandatory. World Neurosurg 2015;84:1838–44.

18. Pallud J, Varlet P, Devaux B, et al. Diffuse low-grade oligodendrogliomas extend beyond MRI-defined abnormalities. Neurology 2010;74:1724–31.

19. Yordanova YN, Duffau H. Supratotal resection of diffuse gliomas—an overview of its multifaceted implications. Neurochirurgie 2017;63:243–9.

20. Yordanova YN, Moritz-Gasser S, Duffau H. Awake surgery for WHO Grade II gliomas within "noneloquent" areas in the left dominant hemisphere: toward a "supratotal" resection. J Neurosurg 2011; 115:232–9.

21. Duffau H. Long-term outcomes after supratotal resection of diffuse low-grade gliomas: a consecutive series with 11-year follow-up. Acta Neurochir (Wien) 2016;158:51–8.

22. Darlix A, Deverdun J, Menjot de Champfleur N, et al. IDH mutation and 1p19q codeletion distinguish two radiological patterns of diffuse low-grade gliomas. J Neurooncol 2017;133:37–45.

23. Zetterling M, Roodakker KR, Berntsson SG, et al. Extension of diffuse low-grade gliomas beyond radiological borders as shown by the coregistration of histopathological and magnetic resonance imaging data. J Neurosurg 2016;125:1155–66.

24. Mandonnet E. Mathematical modeling of low-grade glioma. Bull Acad Natl Med 2011;195:23–34 [in French].

25. Vilasboas T, Herbet G, Duffau H. Challenging the myth of right nondominant hemisphere: lessons from corticosubcortical stimulation mapping in awake surgery and surgical implications. World Neurosurg 2017;103:449–56.

26. Rolland A, Herbet G, Duffau H. Awake surgery for gliomas within the right inferior parietal lobule: new insights into the functional connectivity gained from stimulation mapping and surgical implications. World Neurosurg 2018;112:e393–406.

27. Duffau H. Stimulation mapping of white matter tracts to study brain functional connectivity. Nat Rev Neurol 2015;11:255–65.

28. Teixidor P, Gatignol P, Leroy M, et al. Assessment of verbal working memory before and after surgery for low-grade glioma. J Neurooncol 2007;81: 305–13.

29. Moritz-Gasser S, Herbet G, Duffau H. Mapping the connectivity underlying multimodal (verbal and non-verbal) semantic processing: a brain electrostimulation study. Neuropsychologia 2013;51: 1814–22.

30. Charras P, Herbet G, Deverdun J, et al. Functional reorganization of the attentional networks in low-grade glioma patients: a longitudinal study. Cortex 2015;63:27–41.

31. Lemaitre AL, Herbet G, Duffau H, et al. Preserved metacognitive ability despite unilateral or bilateral anterior prefrontal resection. Brain Cogn 2018;120: 48–57.

32. Mandonnet E, de Witt Hamer P, Pallud J, et al. Silent diffuse low-grade glioma: toward screening and preventive treatment? Cancer 2014;120:1758–62.

33. Duffau H. The huge plastic potential of adult brain and the role of connectomics: new insights provided by serial mappings in glioma surgery. Cortex 2014; 58:325–37.

34. Ius T, Angelini E, Thiebaut de Schotten M, et al. Evidence for potentials and limitations of brain plasticity using an atlas of functional resectability of WHO grade II gliomas: towards a "minimal common brain". NeuroImage 2011;56:992–1000.

35. Herbet G, Maheu M, Costi E, et al. Mapping neuroplastic potential in brain-damaged patients. Brain 2016;139:829–44.

36. Duffau H. A two-level model of interindividual anatomo-functional variability of the brain and its implications for neurosurgery. Cortex 2017;86:303–13.

37. Duffau H. Lessons from brain mapping in surgery for low-grade glioma: insights into associations between tumour and brain plasticity. Lancet Neurol 2005;4:476–86.

38. Southwell DG, Birk HS, Han SJ, et al. Resection of gliomas deemed inoperable by neurosurgeons based on preoperative imaging studies. J Neurosurg 2017; 1–9. https://doi.org/10.3171/2017.5.JNS17166.

39. Ghering K, Sitskoorn MM, Gundy CM, et al. Cognitive rehabilitation in patients with gliomas: a randomized, controlled trial. J Clin Oncol 2009;27:3712–22.

40. Coget A, Deverdun J, Bonafé A, et al. Transient immediate postoperative homotopic functional disconnectivity in low-grade glioma patients. Neuroimage Clin 2018;18:656–62.

41. Boyer A, Deverdun J, Duffau H, et al. Longitudinal changes in cerebellar and thalamic spontaneous neuronal activity after wide-awake surgery of brain tumors: a resting-state fMRI study. Cerebellum 2016;15:451–65.

42. Vassal M, Charroud C, Deverdun J, et al. Recovery of functional connectivity of the sensorimotor network after surgery for diffuse low-grade gliomas involving the supplementary motor area. J Neurosurg 2017;126: 1181–90.

43. Jungk C, Scherer M, Mock A, et al. Prognostic value of the extent of resection in supratentorial WHO grade II astrocytomas stratified for IDH1 mutation status: a single-center volumetric analysis. J Neurooncol 2016;129:319–28.

44. Ahmadi R, Rezvan A, Dictus C, et al. Long-term outcome and survival of surgically treated supratentorial low-grade glioma in adult patients. Acta Neurochir (Wien) 2009;151:1359–65.

45. Martino J, Taillandier L, Moritz-Gasser S, et al. Reoperation is a safe and effective therapeutic strategy in recurrent WHO grade II gliomas within eloquent areas. Acta Neurochir (Wien) 2009;151:427–36.

46. Southwell DG, Hervey-Jumper SL, Perry DW, et al. Intraoperative mapping during repeat awake craniotomy reveals the functional plasticity of adult cortex. J Neurosurg 2016;124:1460–9.

47. Picart T, Herbet G, Moritz-Gasser S, et al. Iterative surgical resections of diffuse glioma with awake mapping: how to deal with cortical plasticity and connectomal constraints? Neurosurgery 2018. https://doi.org/10.1093/neuros/nyy218.

48. Cochereau J, Herbet G, Duffau H. Patients with incidental WHO grade II glioma frequently suffer from neuropsychological disturbances. Acta Neurochir (Wien) 2016;158:305–12.

49. Pallud J, Fontaine D, Duffau H, et al. Natural history of incidental World Health Organization grade II gliomas. Ann Neurol 2010;68:727–33.

50. Shah AH, Madhavan K, Sastry A, et al. Managing intracranial incidental findings suggestive of low-grade glioma: learning from experience. World Neurosurg 2013;80:e75–7.

51. Potts MB, Smith JS, Molinaro AM, et al. Natural history and surgical management of incidentally discovered low-grade gliomas. J Neurosurg 2012; 116:365–72.

52. Almairac F, Herbet G, Moritz-Gasser S, et al. The left inferior fronto-occipital fasciculus subserves language semantics: a multilevel lesion study. Brain Struct Funct 2015;220:1983–95.

53. Herbet G, Lafargue G, Bonnetblanc F, et al. Inferring a dual-stream model of mentalizing from associative white matter fibres disconnection. Brain 2014;137: 944–59.

54. Szalisznyo K, Silverstein DN, Duffau H, et al. Pathological neural attractor dynamics in slowly growing gliomas supports an optimal time frame for white matter plasticity. PLoS One 2013;8:e69798.

55. Cochereau J, Herbet G, Rigau V, et al. Acute progression of untreated incidental WHO Grade II glioma to glioblastoma in an asymptomatic patient. J Neurosurg 2016;124:141–5.

56. Duffau H. Awake surgery for incidental WHO grade II gliomas involving eloquent areas. Acta Neurochir (Wien) 2012;154:575–84.

57. Lima GL, Duffau H. Is there a risk of seizures in "preventive" awake surgery for incidental diffuse low-grade gliomas? J Neurosurg 2015;122:1397–405.

58. Lima GL, Zanello M, Mandonnet E, et al. Incidental diffuse low-grade gliomas: from early detection to preventive neuro-oncological surgery. Neurosurg Rev 2016;39:377–84.

59. Kelly P. Gliomas: survival, origin and early detection. Surg Neurol Int 2010;1:96.

60. Mandonnet E, de Witt Hamer P, Duffau H. MRI screening for glioma: a preliminary survey of healthy potential candidates. Acta Neurochir (Wien) 2016; 158:905–6.

61. Teuber A, Sundermann B, Kugel H, et al. MR imaging of the brain in large cohort studies: feasibility report of the population- and patient-based BiDirect study. Eur Radiol 2017;27:231–8.

62. Morris Z, Whiteley WN, Longstreth WT Jr, et al. Incidental findings on brain magnetic resonance imaging: systematic review and meta-analysis. BMJ 2009;339:b3016.

63. Mandonnet E, Taillandier L, Duffau H. Proposal of screening for diffuse low-grade gliomas in the population from 20 to 40 years. Presse Med 2017;46: 911–20 [in French].

64. Gerin C, Pallud J, Grammaticos B, et al. Improving the time-machine: estimating date of birth of grade II gliomas. Cell Prolif 2012;45:76–90.

65. Mandonnet E, Taillandier L, Duffau H. Proposal of screening for diffuse low-grade gliomas in the population from 20 to 40 years. Presse Med 2017;46: 911–20.

How to Build a Neurosurgical Oncology Practice Specializing in Gliomas

Nader Sanai, MD

KEYWORDS

• Glioma • Mapping • Surgical trials • Fluorescence-guided surgery • Extent of resection

KEY POINTS

- For the neurosurgical oncologist, a specialty practice in gliomas represents an intersection of tailored surgical approaches, emerging intraoperative technologies, expanding surgical trial portfolios, and new paradigms in glioma biology.
- Assembling these disparate pieces into a cohesive career trajectory is a difficult task but ultimately enables the subspecialist to navigate all domains relevant to improving glioma patient outcomes.
- Within the larger clinical and basic science community, thoughtful integration and intensive collaborations are essential mechanisms when building a multidisciplinary glioma program.

INTRODUCTION

In the modern era of glioma management, the neurosurgical oncologist is an essential member of the treatment team and is often the first point of contact for newly diagnosed patients. In most cases, the maximal reduction of tumor burden is an essential first step in the multimodal treatment of low-grade gliomas (LGGs) and high-grade gliomas (HGGs). Central paradigms in the surgical treatment of these tumors include (1) tumor biopsy for histologic diagnosis, (2) cytoreduction to the functional boundaries of the tumor, and (3) judicious application of adjuvant therapy regimens tailored to the clinical circumstances. Increasingly, the neurosurgeon is a key driver of these surgical and nonsurgical treatment options.

Building a subspecialty practice for gliomas is a team effort. Programmatic support for nonsurgical therapies must be developed alongside the capacity for effective operative strategies. Standard neurosurgical techniques, including image-guided surgery, intraoperative stimulation mapping, and fluorescence-guided surgery, are essential but so are advanced neuro-oncology, radiation-oncology, neuroimaging, and neuropathology expertise. Taken together, this treatment team constitutes the de facto primary care physicians for patients with gliomas.

FUNDAMENTALS OF PRACTICE-BUILDING

As in any neurosurgical subspecialty, successful professional development hinges on relationships within the neurosurgical division or department as well as across the community of local and regional physicians. Effective communication, universal availability, and attention to detail are prerequisites for a growing subspecialty practice. Above all, a commitment to advancing patient care must be evident to the physician and patient community.

Department outreach can often be facilitated by existing leadership as well as by personal efforts to work constructively alongside colleagues. Departmental specialization is sometimes mandated but in many cases occurs organically as individual neurosurgeons lead by example. In this regard,

Disclosure: The author has nothing to disclose.
Division of Neurosurgical Oncology, Ivy Brain Tumor Center, Barrow Neurological Institute, 2910 North Third Avenue, Phoenix, AZ 85013, USA
E-mail address: Nader.Sanai@barrowbrainandspine.com

Neurosurg Clin N Am 30 (2019) 129–136
https://doi.org/10.1016/j.nec.2018.08.013

developing a practice specializing in gliomas necessitates referring other cases to colleagues who have demonstrated corresponding subspecialty interests. Ultimately, efforts at subspecialization are optimized when they are approached from the perspective of inclusivity.

Community physician outreach is often as much about availability as education and raising awareness. Glioma patients present to emergency room physicians (after an initial seizure), neurologists (for work-up of neurologic deficits), and family practitioners (due to nonspecific symptoms). Traditional outreach strategies can be effective for this disparate group of clinicians, but the ability for them to connect with a neurosurgeon directly is perhaps more important. The capacity to quickly receive patient information, efficiently intake new patients, and consistently communicate results to referring providers are hallmarks of an effective local outreach program.

Academic visibility is a third pillar of basic practice building for the subspecialty neurosurgeon. Patients with gliomas, particularly at recurrence, are often mobile and well-educated on their disease. Major brain tumor centers with multimodal specialization in the care of gliomas are frequent destinations and often include neurosurgical oncologists who are innovating in this space. Contributions to the literature and participation in both neurosurgical and neuro-oncology conferences not only raise one's profile within the glioma patient and physician community but also ensure early adoption of new investigational technologies, techniques, and therapies.

THE ROLE OF EXTENT OF RESECTION

Principles guiding the appropriate surgical treatment of gliomas include tumor biopsy for histologic diagnosis, cytoreduction within functional boundaries, and carefully considered adjuvant therapies tailored to a patient's clinical condition. The mode of resection for a glioma depends not only on its size and location but also on its anatomy, histologic characteristics, and anticipated sensitivity to adjuvant therapies. A patient's preoperative neurologic and medical conditions also influence the type of operative procedure. An effective glioma specialist tailors surgical approaches to these individual characteristics and considerations. The neurosurgical oncologist has a variety of contemporary neurosurgical methods available (eg, frameless navigational systems, intraoperative imaging, ultrasonography [US], and functional mapping) to achieve an optimal level of cytoreduction of the tumor with minimal postoperative neurologic morbidity.

For glioma patients, controversy persists regarding prognostic factors and treatment options for both low-grade lesions and high-grade lesions. Among the various tumor-related and treatment-related parameters (eg, tumor volume, neurologic status, the timing of surgical intervention, and the use of adjuvant therapy), age and tumor histology are consistently identified as primary predictors of patient prognosis.[1,2] The exact clinical impact of the degree of glioma resection remains, however, unclear, despite meaningful advances in preoperative planning and intraoperative techniques. Glioma resection is critical for tissue diagnosis and decompressing the mass effect of the tumor, yet no class I evidence exists to indicate efficacy based on the extent of the surgical resection. Understanding the effect of surgical resection is important for both LGGs and HGGs despite their differences in biologies, clinical behaviors, and outcomes.

A growing body of reports suggests extensive microsurgical resection is associated with improved life expectancy for patients with LGGs or HGGs.[3] The level of evidence has reached level 2b based on a retrospective analysis of randomized trial data. Most of the evidence, however, is derived from level 3 retrospective case series. Evidence suggests that a more extensive, aggressive resection for LGGs may favorably alter the disease's risk profile for malignant transformation in addition to increasing overall survival.[4] To settle this controversy, a prospective, randomized trial using modern intraoperative techniques and standardized perioperative adjuncts is required. In the absence of such a trial (which may never occur), advances in knowledge must rely on reports from prospective observational studies, retrospective matched studies, and retrospective reviews of randomized trials. An understanding of the existing literature and the nuances of the current evidence supporting the efficacy of the extent of resection is a central quality of any neurosurgical oncologist specializing in gliomas.

EMBRACING INTRAOPERATIVE NEUROSURGICAL TECHNOLOGIES

Over the past 2 decades, the development of advanced neurosurgical imaging technologies, such as intraoperative neuronavigation,[5–10] intraoperative US (iUS),[11–14] and intraoperative MRI (iMRI),[15–23] has improved the potential to achieve complete radiographical resection of a glioma. Frameless intraoperative neuronavigation has gained near-universal implementation at major neurosurgical oncology units in the United States, Europe, and Asia for comparing intraoperative findings with those of preoperative imaging. This tool effectively enables the surgeon to extrapolate the findings of preoperative imaging to 3-D positions within a patient's cranium in real-time. The iUS and iMRI platforms are valuable, but less commonly used, owing to their high costs and, for US, the limited experience among current neurosurgical oncologists.

The clinical utility of various contemporary intraoperative imaging tools, including neuronavigation, iMRI, and iUS, was evaluated in a systematic review of the literature.[24] Collectively, existing studies highlight the need for additional high-quality data and indicate that balancing the use of these complex and expensive intraoperative adjuncts with realistic operative objectives is important. For the neurosurgeon, building a subspecialty practice in gliomas, access to these technologies is greatly facilitative but not essential for a robust practice. As with any technology, its relative value must be evaluated in the context of the practice setting, as well as on the basis of the available evidence.

Low-field iMRI and high-field iMRI enable detailed visualization of the tumor mass and enable real-time interval updates of the 3-D anatomic models used for neuronavigation. During glioma resection, loss of cerebrospinal fluid and tissue edema can result in brain shifts that reduce the accuracy of neuronavigation and thereby impair estimates of the extent and position of residual disease.[25] This challenge provides the rationale for combining iMRI with conventional neuronavigation in guiding glioma surgery. A study involving patients with HGGs, mostly anaplastic astrocytomas,[26] demonstrated the extent of resection can be maximized using low-field-strength iMRI. The use of iMRI also facilitates the surgical treatment of LGG because macroscopic tumor characteristics are unreliable features for distinguishing nonmalignant from malignant tissue. Technical issues with iMRI, however, can lead to image distortion and inaccurate target registration. Moreover, air-tissue interfaces and extravasation of contrast agent due to surgical disruption of the blood-brain barrier can also cause unexpected imaging artifacts. Nevertheless, iMRI is generally effective in maximizing the extent of resection.

Imaging guidance with iUS is a cost-effective and time-efficient alternative to iMRI for use in glioma resection but provides images with low levels of anatomic detail.[27,28] The reductions in the sensitivity and specificity of tumor detection during surgery as a result of imaging artifacts are an important limitation of iUS guidance. Moreover, residual disease less than 1 cm in diameter can be difficult to detect using iUS.[29] Aberrant signals that mimic the appearance of tumor masses can be minimized by placing the transducer directly on the region of interest; however, the cone-shaped field of view can complicate the visualization of superficial cortical lesions located directly deep to the transducer. High-frequency linear probes can provide high-resolution images of tumor tissue and are currently being integrated into the neurosurgical workflow with encouraging results.[30,31]

In both Europe and the United States, fluorescence-guided surgery using 5-aminolevulinic acid (ALA) is increasingly frequent and will soon become an essential technique for any glioma surgeon. The orally administered prodrug 5-ALA can cross the intact blood-brain barrier and is subsequently metabolized intracellularly to form protoporphyrin IX,[32,33] a heme synthesis pathway substrate. Protoporphyrin IX accumulates preferentially in tumor cells and epithelial tissues and emits fluorescence of red-violet light (at wavelengths of 635–704 nm) when excited with blue light (at 400–410 nm wavelengths).[34,35] The neurosurgical integration of 5-ALA–based fluorescence guidance for resection of HGG was demonstrated in a randomized controlled phase IIIa European trial[36]; the trial was terminated after results of an interim analysis in 270 patients revealed the use of 5-ALA–based fluorescence-guided surgery was associated with an increased rate of gross total resection (65% vs 36% for white-light surgery without the use of fluorescence guidance) as well as improved 6-month progression-free survival (41% vs 21.1%). Intraoperative 5-ALA fluorescence is ineffective in guiding the resection of LGGs because such tumors do not typically produce a level of fluorescence visible to the naked eye, although protoporphyrin IX fluorescence in LGG tissue obtained after 5-ALA administration can be measured ex vivo using microscopy.[35,37] Hence, intraoperative confocal microscopy approaches have been developed and used to visualize 5-ALA–based tumor fluorescence in LGGs during microsurgical resection procedures. The United States Food and Drug Administration approved 5-ALA use in 2018, and 5-ALA will soon be available at most major brain tumor centers.

BUILDING AN INTRAOPERATIVE STIMULATION MAPPING PROGRAM

Routinely, glioma patients are at risk of neurologic deficit when planned surgical resections are located within or near functional pathways. Classic anatomic criteria are inadequate in predicting cortical language sites because cortical organization varies considerably between individuals,[38-42] tumor mass effects can distort cerebral topography, and plasticity mechanisms can result in the reorganization of functional networks.[43-48] Thus, for the glioma specialist, intraoperative cortical stimulation remains the standard of care to identify and preserve language function and motor pathways.

An awake craniotomy is recommended for patients with tumors involving the dominant temporal, mid-to-posterior frontal, or mid-to-anterior parietal lobes to identify language sites before excision. Additionally, more complex yet essential cognitive functions (eg, spatial awareness, emotional recognition, and executive functions) can be most effectively monitored and tested using awake craniotomy techniques.[49,50] The necessity for intraoperative testing of these complex functions can often be assessed by conducting a detailed preoperative clinical evaluation of the patient to determine their functional priorities and discuss their expectations following surgery. The use of functional MRI (fMRI) in preoperative assessments might also provide important insights into the location of sensory and motor pathways, is valuable in determining the position of the rolandic cortex.[51] fMRI is unreliable, however, in mapping language sites, and this modality is not an appropriate substitute for intraoperative stimulation mapping.[52] Similarly, somatosensory evoked potential phase-reversal techniques can be used as an adjunct to intraoperative stimulation mapping to identify the location of the primary sensory cortex. This approach involves the use of a strip electrode applied directly to the cortical surface to record evoked electrical activation potential before tumor resection and is associated with a lower risk of intraoperative seizures than cortical stimulation mapping techniques; however, the level of detail somatosensory evoked potential provides is somewhat low, useful only for determining the position of the primary somatosensory cortex.[53]

Development of an intraoperative stimulation mapping program for glioma patients requires the assembly of a multidisciplinary team consisting of a neuroanesthesiologist, a neuropsychologist, an operating room team of nurses and surgical technologists, and a neuroimaging specialist. Often, these local assets already exist but have not yet been unified into a coordinated mapping team. For the neurosurgical oncologist, codifying the stimulation mapping program and educating its members on perioperative and intraoperative protocols are essential first-steps. As in any well-organized health care team, each member must develop a mastery of their individual responsibilities as well as those of their team members. Gold-standard mapping programs, such as those assembled in San Francisco and Montpellier (France),[54,55] indicate that key objectives include less than 2% rates of permanent neurologic deficit and intraoperative seizures. Such efficiency can only be acquired through years of meticulous team-building, thoughtful case selection, and high patient volume.

At the Barrow Neurological Institute, intraoperative mapping cases were scarcely encountered prior to 2011. In the years subsequent, a coordinated, multidisciplinary effort was undertaken to establish and expand an advanced mapping program for patients with eloquent brain tumors. Neurosurgeons, neuroanesthesiologists, operating room nurses, neuropsychologists, and imaging specialists were recruited to contribute to the program. In many instances, these specialists had little to no prior experience with intraoperative stimulation mapping, or the techniques supporting such efforts. General education was provided through formal and informal didactic presentations as well as distribution of both peer-reviewed literature and custom protocols generated for the operating room personnel. Similarly, the authors' patient population, clinic staff, and members of the multidisciplinary tumor board were educated and on-boarded.

Despite comprehensive and institutional efforts, initial results were underwhelming. The learning curve for programmatic success is not driven by individual excellence but rather through collective effort and coordinated process improvement. The metric likely most indicative of an effective system—intraoperative seizure rate—steadily improved from an initial high (**Fig. 1**). This was accomplished through careful postmortem analysis of individual cases as well as cultivation of effective neuroanesthesiologist partners and improved case selection. As a consequence, the proportion of asleep motor mapping cases increased, because the bar was appropriately raised for patients included in awake mapping cases (**Fig. 2**). Taken together, these deliberate modifications, as well as the benefit of time and experience, improved the authors' programmatic results on year-over-year basis. Although the program is still striving to achieve the sub-2% complication rates demonstrated by the standard-bearers in the field, its realization is within reach.

EXPANDING THE SURGICAL TRIALS PORTFOLIO FOR GLIOMAS

Increasingly, surgical trials have proliferated within neurosurgery, particularly within neurosurgical

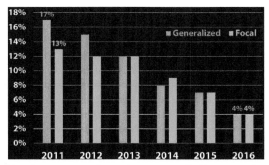

Fig. 1. Intraoperative seizure rates decline over the first 5 years of a newly developed intraoperative mapping program.

oncology. For the neurosurgical oncologist treating gliomas, the importance of developing more effective adjuvant therapies is self-evident. Most patients, however, complete the surgical phase of their treatment and are subsequently enrolled in clinical trials beyond the scope of their neurosurgical care.[56] The current rise of surgical trials in neuro-oncology, however, unify the clinical and investigational teams by beginning the investigational process during the perioperative period. In this context, the neurosurgical oncologist is less of a passive participant in the trial and, in many cases, becomes an essential team member for the surgical phase of the study as well as the study design and patient accrual stages.[57]

Beyond conventional device development, surgical trials are now a valued component of modern adjuvant therapy studies. Phase 0 clinical trials, for example, identify promising new drugs by humanizing preclinical studies. Unlike non–central nervous system cancer studies, where interventional radiologists can provide safe access to tissue samples at multiple time points, tissue-based studies in neuro-oncology depend on a partnership with a neurosurgical specialist. Especially

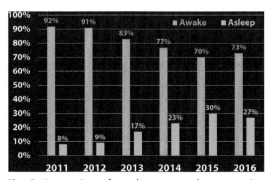

Fig. 2. Proportion of awake versus asleep mapping cases over the first 5 years of a newly developed intraoperative mapping program.

for phase 0 studies, high levels of technical stringency and multidisciplinary coordination are required to obtain reliable data. The neurosurgical oncologist, therefore, plays an important role in both patient selection and study consent. Intraoperatively, stringent protocols for timed tissue collection also require careful coordination of the operating room staff and neurosurgical team. Thus, operating room logistics and issues of surgical timing play an essential role in determining whether the sample collection parameters of the study can be met. For the neurosurgical oncologist, the logistical challenges of the phase 0 study patient can be overcome through careful coordination with the operating room staff (including neuroanesthesiologists, nurses, and surgical technologists) as well as thoughtful case scheduling to avoid delays and diversions routinely encountered in the operating room. Taken together, these perioperative and intraoperative responsibilities position the neurosurgical oncologist as one of several key members of the modern glioma clinical trials team.

INTEGRATING THE BASIC SCIENCE OF GLIOMAS

The need for a better understanding of glioma biology is a universally recognized reality of the field. Tomorrow's glioma specialists must be as comfortable considering surgical approaches as they are discussing the tumor genetics that currently drive adjuvant decision-making. The recent transition to a molecular classification system for the World Health Organization grading exemplifies this transition and new reality. Clinical trials are increasingly predicated on genetic entry criteria, and clinical decision making is often influenced by prognostic and predictive biomarkers. Even with respect to the extent of resection, evidence suggests molecular features, such as isocitrate dehydrogenase mutation status, may be a necessary consideration when planning HGG surgery.[58] For the neurosurgeon/neuroscientist, the need for dual expertise is a natural extension of this career model. Even for the purely clinical neurosurgical oncologist, however, an in-depth awareness of the molecular neuro-oncology and its steady evolution is a necessity for effective practice. This can be accomplished through the development of habits in reading the neuroscience literature, attending nonsurgical neuro-oncology meetings, and participating in local and consortium clinical trials. A close working relationship with colleagues in clinical neuro-oncology, neuro-radiation oncology, and neuropathology also facilitates this knowledge base.

SUMMARY

Building a subspecialty practice in gliomas re-quires a multimodal approach to neurosurgery, including an understanding of basic practice-building methods, a nuanced approach to the extent of resection, early adoption of neurosur-gical technologies, direct engagement of clinical trials, and a comfortable relationship with glioma biology. Although the management of glioma pa-tients remains an uphill battle, neurosurgical on-cologists who can successfully navigate these opportunities will undoubtedly yield the finest re-sults as well as place their patients in the best possible condition to outperform the disease.

ACKNOWLEDGMENTS

The author is indebted to John Essex (Peak Medical Editing) for copy editing.

REFERENCES

1. Sanai N, Berger MS. Glioma extent of resection and its impact on patient outcome. Neurosurgery 2008; 62(4):753–64 [discussion: 264–756].

2. Sanai N, Chang S, Berger MS. Low-grade gliomas in adults. J Neurosurg 2011;115(5):948–65.

3. Hardesty DA, Sanai N. The value of glioma extent of resection in the modern neurosurgical era. Front Neurol 2012;3:140.

4. Smith JS, Chang EF, Lamborn KR, et al. Role of extent of resection in the long-term outcome of low-grade hemispheric gliomas. J Clin Oncol 2008; 26(8):1338–45.

5. Warnke PC. Stereotactic volumetric resection of gli-omas. Acta Neurochir Suppl 2003;88:5–8.

6. Krishnan R, Raabe A, Hattingen E, et al. Functional magnetic resonance imaging-integrated neuronavi-gation: correlation between lesion-to-motor cortex distance and outcome. Neurosurgery 2004;55(4): 904–14 [discusssion: 914–5].

7. Wu JS, Zhou LF, Tang WJ, et al. Clinical evaluation and follow-up outcome of diffusion tensor imaging-based functional neuronavigation: a prospective, controlled study in patients with gliomas involving pyramidal tracts. Neurosurgery 2007;61(5):935–48 [discussion: 948–9].

8. Reithmeier T, Krammer M, Gumprecht H, et al. Neu-ronavigation combined with electrophysiological monitoring for surgery of lesions in eloquent brain areas in 42 cases: a retrospective comparison of the neurological outcome and the quality of resec-tion with a control group with similar lesions. Minim Invasive Neurosurg 2003;46(2):65–71.

9. Kurimoto M, Hayashi N, Kamiyama H, et al. Impact of neuronavigation and image-guided extensive resection for adult patients with supratentorial malignant astrocytomas: a single-institution retro-spective study. Minim Invasive Neurosurg 2004; 47(5):278–83.

10. Willems PW, Taphoorn MJ, Burger H, et al. Effective-ness of neuronavigation in resecting solitary intrace-rebral contrast-enhancing tumors: a randomized controlled trial. J Neurosurg 2006;104(3):360–8.

11. Unsgaard G, Selbekk T, Brostrup Muller T, et al. Abil-ity of navigated 3D ultrasound to delineate gliomas and metastases–comparison of image interpreta-tions with histopathology. Acta Neurochir (Wien) 2005;147(12):1259–69 [discussion: 1269].

12. Coenen VA, Krings T, Weidemann J, et al. Sequential visualization of brain and fiber tract deformation dur-ing intracranial surgery with three-dimensional ultra-sound: an approach to evaluate the effect of brain shift. Neurosurgery 2005;56(1 Suppl):133–41 [dis-cussion: 133–41].

13. Reinacher PC, van Velthoven V. Intraoperative ultra-sound imaging: practical applicability as a real-time navigation system. Acta Neurochir Suppl 2003;85: 89–93.

14. Nikas DC, Hartov A, Lunn K, et al. Coregistered in-traoperative ultrasonography in resection of malig-nant glioma. Neurosurg Focus 2003;14(2):e6.

15. Senft C, Seifert V, Hermann E, et al. Usefulness of in-traoperative ultra low-field magnetic resonance im-aging in glioma surgery. Neurosurgery 2008;63(4 Suppl 2):257–66 [discussion 266–57].

16. Nimsky C, Fujita A, Ganslandt O, et al. Volumetric assessment of glioma removal by intraoperative high-field magnetic resonance imaging. Neurosur-gery 2004;55(2):358–70 [discussion: 370–51].

17. Hall WA, Liu H, Maxwell RE, et al. Influence of 1.5-Tesla intraoperative MR imaging on surgical deci-sion making. Acta Neurochir Suppl 2003;85:29–37.

18. Hirschberg H, Samset E, Hol PK, et al. Impact of intra-operative MRI on the surgical results for high-grade gliomas. Minim Invasive Neurosurg 2005;48(2):77–84.

19. Senft C, Bink A, Heckelmann M, et al. Glioma extent of resection and ultra-low-field iMRI: interim analysis of a prospective randomized trial. Acta Neurochir Suppl 2011;109:49–53.

20. Hatiboglu MA, Weinberg JS, Suki D, et al. Impact of intraoperative high-field magnetic resonance imag-ing guidance on glioma surgery: a prospective volu-metric analysis. Neurosurgery 2009;64(6):1073–81 [discussion: 1081].

21. Pamir MN, Ozduman K, Dincer A, et al. First intrao-perative, shared-resource, ultrahigh-field 3-Tesla magnetic resonance imaging system and its appli-cation in low-grade glioma resection. J Neurosurg 2010;112(1):57–69.

22. Black PM, Alexander E 3rd, Martin C, et al. Crani-otomy for tumor treatment in an intraoperative mag-netic resonance imaging unit. Neurosurgery 1999; 45(3):423–31 [discussion: 431–23].

23. Claus EB, Horlacher A, Hsu L, et al. Survival rates in patients with low-grade glioma after intraoperative magnetic resonance image guidance. Cancer 2005;103(6):1227–33.

24. Barone DG, Lawrie TA, Hart MG. Image guided surgery for the resection of brain tumours. Cochrane Database Syst Rev 2014;(1):CD009685.

25. Nimsky C, Ganslandt O, Tomandl B, et al. Low-field magnetic resonance imaging for intraoperative use in neurosurgery: a 5-year experience. Eur Radiol 2002;12(11):2690–703.

26. Muragaki Y, Iseki H, Maruyama T, et al. Information-guided surgical management of gliomas using low-field-strength intraoperative MRI. Acta Neurochir Suppl 2011;109:67–72.

27. Chandler WF, Knake JE, McGillicuddy JE, et al. Intraoperative use of real-time ultrasonography in neurosurgery. J Neurosurg 1982;57(2):157–63.

28. Prada F, Perin A, Martegani A, et al. Intraoperative contrast-enhanced ultrasound for brain tumor surgery. Neurosurgery 2014;74(5):542–52 [discussion: 552].

29. Gerganov VM, Samii A, Akbarian A, et al. Reliability of intraoperative high-resolution 2D ultrasound as an alternative to high-field strength MR imaging for tumor resection control: a prospective comparative study. J Neurosurg 2009;111(3):512–9.

30. Coburger J, Konig RW, Scheuerle A, et al. Navigated high frequency ultrasound: description of technique and clinical comparison with conventional intracranial ultrasound. World Neurosurg 2014;82(3–4):366–75.

31. Solheim O, Selbekk T, Jakola AS, et al. Ultrasound-guided operations in unselected high-grade gliomas–overall results, impact of image quality and patient selection. Acta Neurochir (Wien) 2010;152(11):1873–86.

32. Stummer W, Stepp H, Moller G, et al. Technical principles for protoporphyrin-IX-fluorescence guided microsurgical resection of malignant glioma tissue. Acta Neurochir (Wien) 1998;140(10):995–1000.

33. Duffner F, Ritz R, Freudenstein D, et al. Specific intensity imaging for glioblastoma and neural cell cultures with 5-aminolevulinic acid-derived protoporphyrin IX. J Neurooncol 2005;71(2):107–11.

34. Stummer W, Reulen HJ, Novotny A, et al. Fluorescence-guided resections of malignant gliomas–an overview. Acta Neurochir Suppl 2003;88:9–12.

35. Ishihara R, Katayama Y, Watanabe T, et al. Quantitative spectroscopic analysis of 5-aminolevulinic acid-induced protoporphyrin IX fluorescence intensity in diffusely infiltrating astrocytomas. Neurol Med Chir (Tokyo) 2007;47(2):53–7 [discussion: 57].

36. Stummer W, Pichlmeier U, Meinel T, et al. Fluorescence-guided surgery with 5-aminolevulinic acid for resection of malignant glioma: a randomised controlled multicentre phase III trial. Lancet Oncol 2006;7(5):392–401.

37. Floeth FW, Sabel M, Ewelt C, et al. Comparison of (18)F-FET PET and 5-ALA fluorescence in cerebral gliomas. Eur J Nucl Med Mol Imaging 2011;38(4):731–41.

38. Herholz K, Thiel A, Wienhard K, et al. Individual functional anatomy of verb generation. Neuroimage 1996;3(3 Pt 1):185–94.

39. Ojemann G, Ojemann J, Lettich E, et al. Cortical language localization in left, dominant hemisphere. An electrical stimulation mapping investigation in 117 patients. J Neurosurg 1989;71(3):316–26.

40. Ojemann GA, Whitaker HA. Language localization and variability. Brain Lang 1978;6(2):239–60.

41. Ojemann GA. Individual variability in cortical localization of language. J Neurosurg 1979;50(2):164–9.

42. Glasser MF, Coalson TS, Robinson EC, et al. A multimodal parcellation of human cerebral cortex. Nature 2016;536(7615):171–8.

43. Ojemann JG, Miller JW, Silbergeld DL. Preserved function in brain invaded by tumor. Neurosurgery 1996;39(2):253–8 [discussion: 258–9].

44. Seitz RJ, Huang Y, Knorr U, et al. Large-scale plasticity of the human motor cortex. Neuroreport 1995;6(5):742–4.

45. Wunderlich G, Knorr U, Herzog H, et al. Precentral glioma location determines the displacement of cortical hand representation. Neurosurgery 1998;42(1):18–26 [discussion: 26–7].

46. Robles SG, Gatignol P, Lehericy S, et al. Long-term brain plasticity allowing a multistage surgical approach to World Health Organization Grade II gliomas in eloquent areas. J Neurosurg 2008;109(4):615–24.

47. Duffau H. Brain plasticity: from pathophysiological mechanisms to therapeutic applications. J Clin Neurosci 2006;13(9):885–97.

48. Duffau H, Taillandier L, Gatignol P, et al. The insular lobe and brain plasticity: lessons from tumor surgery. Clin Neurol Neurosurg 2006;108(6):543–8.

49. Duffau H. Stimulation mapping of white matter tracts to study brain functional connectivity. Nat Rev Neurol 2015;11(5):255–65.

50. Moritz-Gasser S, Herbet G, Maldonado IL, et al. Lexical access speed is significantly correlated with the return to professional activities after awake surgery for low-grade gliomas. J Neurooncol 2012;107(3):633–41.

51. Wengenroth M, Blatow M, Guenther J, et al. Diagnostic benefits of presurgical fMRI in patients with brain tumours in the primary sensorimotor cortex. Eur Radiol 2011;21(7):1517–25.

52. Cochereau J, Deverdun J, Herbet G, et al. Comparison between resting state fMRI networks and responsive cortical stimulations in glioma patients. Hum Brain Mapp 2016;37(11):3721–32.

53. Romstock J, Fahlbusch R, Ganslandt O, et al. Localisation of the sensorimotor cortex during surgery for

brain tumours: feasibility and waveform patterns of somatosensory evoked potentials. J Neurol Neurosurg Psychiatry 2002;72(2):221–9.

54. Sanai N, Mirzadeh Z, Berger MS. Functional outcome after language mapping for glioma resection. N Engl J Med 2008;358(1):18–27.

55. Duffau H, Capelle L, Denvil D, et al. Usefulness of intraoperative electrical subcortical mapping during surgery for low-grade gliomas located within eloquent brain regions: functional results in a consecutive series of 103 patients. J Neurosurg 2003;98(4):764–78.

56. Lang FF, Asher A. Prospective clinical trials of brain tumor therapy: the critical role of neurosurgeons. J Neurooncol 2004;69(1–3):151–67.

57. Lang FF, Gilbert MR, Puduvalli VK, et al. Toward better early-phase brain tumor clinical trials: a reappraisal of current methods and proposals for future strategies. Neuro Oncol 2002;4(4):268–77.

58. Beiko J, Suki D, Hess KR, et al. IDH1 mutant malignant astrocytomas are more amenable to surgical resection and have a survival benefit associated with maximal surgical resection. Neuro Oncol 2014;16(1):81–91.

Moving?

Make sure your subscription moves with you!

To notify us of your new address, find your **Clinics Account Number** (located on your mailing label above your name), and contact customer service at:

Email: journalscustomerservice-usa@elsevier.com

800-654-2452 (subscribers in the U.S. & Canada)
314-447-8871 (subscribers outside of the U.S. & Canada)

Fax number: 314-447-8029

Elsevier Health Sciences Division
Subscription Customer Service
3251 Riverport Lane
Maryland Heights, MO 63043

Printed and bound by CPI Group (UK) Ltd, Croydon, CR0 4YY

08/05/2025

01864741-0007